"Food offerings are a universal gesture to show care and support. This workbook highlights a simple formula connecting what we eat to how we feel. It's especially important during times of high stress. I often suggest ways for parents in the child welfare system to use food as a tool so they can be at their best. I personally use protein for my wellness, performance anxiety, and afternoon fatigue."

—**Ambrosia Eberhardt**, family impact statewide manager for the Parents for Parents program at the Children's Home Society of Washington; and board member and founding member of the International Parent Advocacy Network

"This is a well-, thoughtfully laid out workbook that profoundly benefits and encourages individuals struggling with anxiety, post-traumatic stress disorder (PTSD), and fatigue. The reader develops a clear, applicable understanding of relevant neuroscience and physiology while acquiring an effective toolbox to improve quality of life. Each chapter and the appendix provide accessible how-tos, charts, menus, experiments—all designed to accommodate a busy lifestyle and reduce anxiety. A must-read!"

—**Andrea St. Clair, MA, SUDP**, positive alternative client care coordinator

"This is a must-read for all clinicians helping clients' access healthy coping skills. After applying this information in my clinical practice, many of my clients have eliminated or significantly reduced panic attacks, anxiety, irritability, and depression; and improved their relationships. I engage all of my clients in the three-day protein experiment. I love hearing them say, 'The lizard snacks worked!'"

—**Yesenia C. Dominguez, LCSW, PPSC**, clinical social worker providing direct services to migrant, Latinx community members of various ages in Southern California

"In my clinical practice, I have witnessed a sharp increase in anxiety over the last decade, specifically the last few years. The strategies in *Fuel Your Brain, Not Your Anxiety* have been essential additions to the interventions I create with my clients. Using these interventions, my clients have been able to build strong, healthy foundations. And with a strong foundation, my clients are better equipped to weather the continual storms of life."

—**Jeanne F. MSW, LICSW**, clinical social worker practicing for over twenty years, working with a diverse demographic of adults, teens, and couples; and owner of Practical Therapy, LLC

"Life-changing. This is not an exaggeration of what will happen when you read this workbook. The authors have created tools for resolving the overwhelm and fatigue that many of us feel. In court, families in crisis need a judicial officer who is thoughtful and responsive when making decisions that dramatically impact their lives. Returning home after listening to traumatic events and making complex decisions, my family still needs a present and creative person. This workbook fulfills those intentions and so much more."

—**Michelle Ressa, JD**, Washington superior court commissioner, adjunct professor at Gonzaga University School of Law, advisory board member to Catholic Charities of Eastern Washington for Rising Strong, and board member of Family Impact Network

"I have witnessed Kristen Allott work with busy CEOs and senior leadership teams, giving them the tools they need to make better decisions throughout their days. Kristen explains what is happening in our brains with simple, understandable concepts, and follows this up with easy-to-implement solutions. Kristen's work has helped numerous leaders lead more fulfilling lives with much less stress and chaos!"

—**Mike Huse**, master chair of Vistage-Seattle, the world's largest network of CEOs; and past president, COO, and vice president of operations for Quality Food Center (QFC)

"The authors offer their extensive experience with clarity and compassion, in formats that excite readers to make doable changes for significant impacts. Their unique approach empowers readers to embody a practical understanding of the physiological relationship between body, food, and mental health. They guide readers towards gains in self-knowledge that translate to more mindful choices. This workbook intelligently addresses the challenges of modern lifestyles, providing simple, everyday changes that become the backbone for living a more fulfilling life."

> —**Christine and Po Karczewski**, holistic psychiatric advanced registered nurse practitioners (ARNPs); cofounders of Mount Tahoma Sanctuary and The Healing Field in Tacoma, WA; and activists for a mental health paradigm shift

"*Fuel Your Brain, Not Your Anxiety* brings the power of science, along with concrete examples of behavioral changes, into an easy-to-understand approach that supports long-term sobriety. At our treatment center, countless clients have benefited from this program. Through embracing the direct and clearly described concepts, our clients found their resulting behavior changes made a big difference in their mood and overall well-being. A great read that belongs on everyone's shelf who has a commitment to their own and their client's well-being."

> —**Amy Condon, MA**, current clinical director at A Positive Alternative Treatment Program in Seattle, WA; and licensed chemical dependency professional and certified counselor with the State of Washington

"Kristen Allott and Natasha Duarte present a revolutionary and completely accessible way for all folks to influence their own mental health. They illustrate the impact our daily choices can have; and the illustration is not only with words, but also imagery and tables to help us step-by-step, to step into a better expression of ourselves. My only question is, 'When's the app going to be released?!'"

> —**Amy C. Darling, LAc, MAcOM**, clinical acupuncturist, herbalist, health educator, and Zen student

Fuel Your Brain, Not Your Anxiety

Stop the Cycle of Worry, Fatigue & Sugar Cravings with Simple Protein-Rich Foods

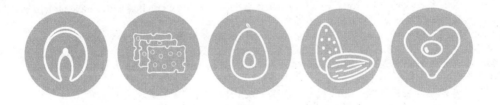

Kristen Allott, ND, MS • Natasha Duarte, MS

New Harbinger Publications, Inc.

Publisher's Note

The material in this book is for educational purposes only, and is intended to supplement, not replace, the advice of a trained health professional. As with all new diet and nutritional regimens, the program described in this book should be followed only after first consulting with your health professional, to make sure it is appropriate for your individual circumstances. If you know or suspect that you have a health problem, you should consult with a health professional. The authors and the publisher expressly disclaim responsibility for any adverse effects that may result from the use or application of the information contained in this book.

Distributed in Canada by Raincoast Books

Copyright © 2021 by Kristen Allott and Natasha Duarte
New Harbinger Publications, Inc.
5674 Shattuck Avenue
Oakland, CA 94609
www.newharbinger.com

The brain image used in the "What Is Your Power Supply?" figure and others is made by Smashicons from http://www.flaticon.com.

Cover design by Amy Daniel

Acquired by Jess O'Brien

Edited by Gretel Hakanson

Library of Congress Cataloging-in-Publication Data

Names: Allott, Kristen, author. | Duarte, Natasha, author.
Title: Fuel your brain, not your anxiety : stop the cycle of worry, fatigue, and sugar cravings with simple protein-rich foods / Kristen Allott, Natasha Duarte.
Description: Oakland, CA : New Harbinger Publications, [2021] | Includes bibliographical references.
Identifiers: LCCN 2020033222 (print) | LCCN 2020033223 (ebook) | ISBN 9781684036233 (trade paperback) | ISBN 9781684036240 (pdf) | ISBN 9781684036257 (epub)
Subjects: LCSH: Brain. | Nutrition. | Diet. | Self-care, Health.
Classification: LCC QP376 .A4235 2021 (print) | LCC QP376 (ebook) | DDC 612.8/2--dc23
LC record available at https://lccn.loc.gov/2020033222
LC ebook record available at https://lccn.loc.gov/2020033223

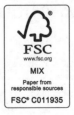
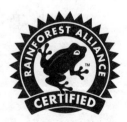

Printed in the United States of America

23   22   21

10   9   8   7   6   5   4   3   2   1   First Printing

Contents

Foreword

I remember my first big public talk at a professional conference during graduate school. My anxiety was almost overwhelming as I waited to present my research in an auditorium full of graduate students, professors, and professional practitioners. As I waited my turn to present, I began to question my goals. The anxiety was taking over as I began to sweat and feel my heart beating faster. My mind was racing and I was suddenly unsure of what I was going to say during my talk.

During graduate school, one of my goals included becoming a professor at a major research university. In order to accomplish this, I would have to actively publish research in scientific journals and speak publicly at professional conferences. It would be a normal part of this life. Ultimately, I progressed through graduate education and became a full professor with tenure at a major research institution. This journey required me to speak publicly at countless conferences. To this day, the very idea of public speaking creates moments of anxiety, stress, and worry. Do we have the ability to control this anxiety through diet and exercise?

My research is focused on hope as a coping resource for those experiencing stress and adversity associated with trauma. Hope is based upon our future expectation of achieving desirable goals. In order to be hopeful, you must be able to identify pathways (mental road maps) to those goals, conceiving and overcoming the potential barriers you might experience. This is referred to as pathways thinking. We must also possess the willpower (mental energy) necessary to pursue these pathways. Willpower is the motivational driver of our ability to hope.

In this powerful workbook, Kristen and Natasha have done a wonderful job providing tools to maintain willpower. This workbook will give you step-by-step strategies to change your life through healthy diet, sleep, and simple exercise.

Among all the positive outcomes associated with having hope, at least two findings are specific to the wonderful workbook you hold in your hands. First, this workbook uses the science of hope by offering pathways to reduce your anxiety and improve your mental clarity and energy. The second is that your willpower—the motivational force behind hope—is connected to your power supply, which is determined in part by what and when you eat. Nutrition matters in the science of hope! Hope is one of the best predictors of your capacity to thrive; your well-being depends on your ability to hope.

This workbook walks you through strategies to stabilize your glucose levels with protein-rich foods, effectively understand food labels, feel the impact of movement and sleep, and connect with your health care provider, all in an effort to improve your well-being. Kristen and Natasha have taken the extraordinary step of making an interactive workbook that gives you the tools to take control of reducing your anxiety and make hope rise.

—Chan M. Hellman, PhD
Professor and director, Hope Research Center at the
University of Oklahoma, Tulsa
Coauthor of *HOPE Rising: How The Science of HOPE
Can Change Your Life*

Introduction

If you picked up this book, you've probably experienced anxiety, worry, or fatigue that has limited your life and you're wondering if you have all the tools you need. Anxiety is complex; it's that felt sense of nervousness when our hearts and thoughts race, our energy and mental clarity recede, and we're more reactive than responsive to what's occurring. We need some anxiety to keep us alive, and it can motivate us; however, in too large of a dose, anxiety can paralyze us and limit our world. Part of the complexity of anxiety is that it's embedded in everyone's personal story, so why and how it shows up is different for each person. For every story of anxiety, there is an emotional component and a physical or physiological component.

Scientific studies are changing our thinking about emotions, about why certain emotional patterns emerge for each of us, and about how we regulate or perhaps struggle with regulating them. Anxiety is an important emotion. It's accompanied by specific thought patterns and can also be accompanied by physical symptoms. However, "anxiety" is also an umbrella term. In other words, not everyone's anxiety is the same. Anxiety can exist in our minds, in our brains, in our bodies, and also within our relationships. This means that in order to manage anxiety, it's essential to define the details that are unique to you.

In this workbook, we approach understanding our own and other people's anxiety by looking at four quadrants of a person: the body, the brain, relationships, and the mind. We consider these four quadrants because they are usually the most affected by anxiety and fatigue and they play an important role in supporting our overall well-being.

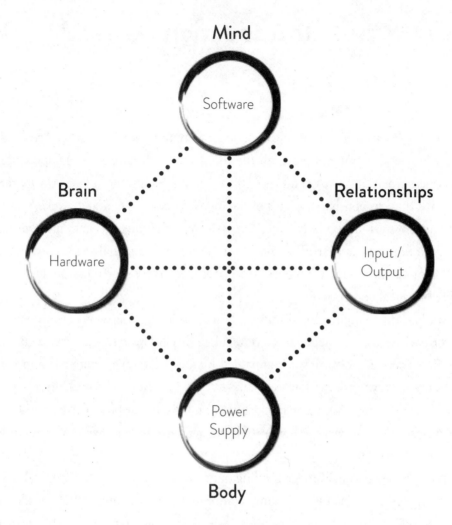

The Four Quadrants of Self

First, there's the *body*. When we provide our body with what it needs, ensuring that it has a sufficient power supply, we are not just supporting our physical health. We are also supporting our brain health, which is necessary for decision making, creativity, and our ability to use emotions to understand who we are. Additionally, when we have a well-fueled and cared-for body, we have the energy to enjoy our lives, engage in meaningful work, and seek new adventures.

Then there's the *brain*. The brain is a very complex organ that works to filter the information from our senses to keep us alive. Different parts of the brain determine how we experience the world. The power supply from the body influences which part of the brain is filtering the information coming to us about our world. For simplicity, we are going to talk about the brain in two modes: the "responsive-cortex brain" and the "reactive-limbic brain."

When we feel safe, relaxed, and well fed, the input derived from sensing our world travels to higher-functioning parts of the brain: the *cerebral cortex* and the *hippocampus*. These parts of the brain enable us to make clear and sound decisions, even amid complex situations and problems. When you're in your responsive-cortex brain, you're conscious, able to learn, and able to make appropriate and creative decisions based on both past experiences and present information.

By contrast, when we feel unsafe, stressed, or underfed, the body releases adrenaline. When the brain is exposed to adrenaline, sensory input stops traveling primarily to the responsive-cortex brain and is instead routed to the reactive-limbic brain. Once the reactive-limbic part of the brain becomes the primary recipient of sensory input, it's forced to choose from the four instinctual reactions: *fight*, *flight*, *freeze or disappear*, and *default to a habit or the past*.

Historically, say, ten thousand years ago, we might have eaten only once a day and could operate from our habitual, reactive-limbic brain most of the day because it served us well. We would get up and seek food or shelter and interact with our family and community in predictable patterns. There was a lot of routine to the day. The demands of our lives today are significantly different. We're almost always responding to new information, relating to community through text, email, or social media, and especially for those whose work involves processing and analyzing information, we're asked to be creative all the time.

Our bodies' power supplies are challenged daily by the timing and types of food we eat and our lack of routines, which in turn limit the amount of fuel reaching our brains. The instability of the power supply for our bodies and brains increases the frequency at which we're thinking through our reactive-limbic brain, which increases anxiety, worry, and fatigue. The focus of this workbook is to improve your power supply from your body to your brain—most prominently, by introducing protein more frequently into your diet—so your responsive-cortex brain is engaged more consistently and you spend less time in your reactive-limbic brain. This means that you'll be less anxious and have more energy to engage in your life.

Relationships can also influence the amount and frequency of your anxiety. By "relationships," we mean the input to and output from the brain. The term encompasses the relationships we have with people around us as well as the environments in which we live and our connection to nature. Some relationships are stable, caring, and safe. These relationships lower anxiety because they support us through whatever is happening. Other relationships can be challenging, unstable, or unsafe. These are harder to manage, causing heightened anxiety, worry, and fatigue. The brain demands more fuel just to be in these relationships, which means that the body is more likely to crave foods high in carbohydrates. The sense of anxiety in these relationships is often a roller coaster, which drains our power supply, decreasing our energy, mental clarity, and sense of resiliency.

The fourth area is *the mind*. Dr. Dan Siegel (2010) explains that the mind is an emergent property that arises from the brain, the body, and the relationships we're in. You may be asking yourself, *What is an emergent property?* Clouds are emergent properties. If you have ever been caught in a rainstorm, you believe in clouds. However, they exist only when there is the right combination of water, wind, and air pressure. If you go up into the sky in a plane and stick a box out the window, you can't put clouds into the box. Our minds are the same way: when our bodies, brains, and relationships are working together, our minds will form. Another way to think about this is to consider when a coworker is super-sick with the flu. Part of why they get sent home is because they are too fatigued, and in that moment, their particular combination of brain-body-relationships cannot support "a mind" that's functional at work.

When the mind is clear, we have curiosity about ourselves and others versus judgment. A clear mind leads to a compassionate observational self. This is the curious responsive-cortex brain part that if we make a mistake, we might ask, "Why did I just do that?" In contrast, a reactive-limbic brain would say something like, "Why are you so dumb that you did that?" You might call the mean voice in your head the Inner Critic. Of course, it's just your brain trying to keep you safe, but because the Inner Critic is always pushing you, the reactive-limbic brain can make you very anxious. The Inner Critic can also put you in what some call the "prison of perfection." Personally, we prefer the calmness of the responsive-cortex brain and the curious mind.

Ultimately, understanding the cause of your anxiety (often, factors like having overwhelming events happen to you as a child, having a history of trauma or abuse, doing something new or unknown and therefore stressful, or experiencing events that will change the course of your life, to name a few) and understanding where your anxiety is coming from—the body, brain, relationships, or mind—is helpful in determining how to treat it. And because everything that happens in any of the quadrants affects the others, treating the cause of anxiety in one area will have a ripple effect.

Often, the circumstances that commonly provoke anxiety—those big life changes or pivotal past events—will make you emotionally anxious, and your inner dialogue can make the situation or your life in general so much more challenging. One approach for treating these causes of anxiety is to work with a therapist. Most therapies (and most books about anxiety) focus on the connection between the mind and brain, the internal dialogue, and healing the past so it doesn't impact our lives so heavily. Some therapies, such as CBT (cognitive behavioral therapy) and DBT (dialectical behavioral therapy), provide additional emotional skills, such as mindfulness, that you may have heard of or tried before. Another approach to treating anxiety is through pharmaceutical intervention, where a prescriber, such as a medical doctor or psychiatric nurse practitioner, prescribes a medication to lower your anxiety. Medications can help stabilize the brain while you try to address the historic or inner dialogue that's driving anxiety.

What is not addressed through therapy or medication is your physiology, which is why this book focuses on a third option—the protein solution to anxiety. Anxiety can be created or accelerated by what is happening to the power supply for the body. By assuring that the brain has fuel, nutrients, and resources to function optimally, the symptoms of anxiety can be reduced anywhere from 10 to 50 percent. Additionally, it's exhausting to be anxious, so implementing the protein solution can also improve fatigue by anywhere from 10 to 50 percent.

In this book, we'll review the science of protein consumption and glucose regulation—the process by which glucose levels are maintained in your bloodstream, which is vastly improved when you incorporate more protein into your diet. We'll also introduce you to a woman named Luca who's struggling with some of the same things you're probably struggling with, as she navigates family and work life. You may be able to identify with the patterns Luca experiences and see how the physiology plays out in her life. Understanding the physiology will help you understand the *why* behind your symptoms. And when you understand that, it will be easier to know *when* and *how* to use the tools we'll teach you to slow down or stop anxiety, worry, and fatigue.

WHO THIS WORKBOOK IS FOR

This book is for you if you have any of the following:

- General anxiety or panic attacks

- Specific anxiety: phobias, performance anxiety, social anxiety, obsessive-compulsive disorder, or anxiety around high-stakes decision making

- Early-morning waking, waking with anxiety or irritation, or not being able to wake up in the morning

- Symptoms of post-traumatic stress disorder (PTSD), including nightmares and night terrors

- Sugar cravings

- Fatigue in general, and afternoon fatigue specifically

Even though everyone experiences anxiety differently, the basic physiological process of how your brain is fueled is common to every human. If you have a brain and a body, the tools presented in this workbook will help. Kristen, in her capacity as a naturopathic physician, teaches these tools to a wide range of individuals—all wanting to have less anxiety and worry and more energy and mental clarity. In her clinical practice, she routinely sees a drop in anxiety of at least 20 percent. What that means on a scale of 1 to 10, where 1 is no anxiety at all and 10 is a full-blown panic attack, is that a person regularly hitting a 9 can drop their anxiety level to a 7 simply by making achievable changes to diet. Granted, a 7 is still pretty anxious, but it's a low enough level of anxiety that people can then access and use other emotion-based tools. Some people who started using protein solutions have found their symptoms reduced by as much as 50 percent. Fundamentally, the amount of relief you might get depends on how much of your anxiety is due to physical causes and how much is from emotional causes. This workbook will help you better understand the physical causes. After trying the strategies outlined, you may decide they help so much that you will use them almost every day, or you may decide to use them as tools for specific occasions.

Our goal in this book is to give you a new way to think about what is driving your anxiety and new tools to reduce your anxiety as well as increase your energy and mental clarity. With each tool we introduce, we'll provide experiments you can try—an activity, a specific amount of time to dedicate to it (from 30 seconds to 45 days), and a sense of what the possible outcomes might be—so you can practice using the tools and see if and how they impact your symptoms. These experiments are opportunities to learn about yourself and your body. They're a way of trying something new with the intention of noticing whether the new behavior makes you feel better or not. We think experiments are the best way to know how something will affect your experience in your body and mind. All in all, as you work through the workbook, you'll develop a better picture of what's happening for you, and this will help you have a new framework to explain why and when it's happening and what to do about it.

WHAT YOU'LL FIND IN THIS WORKBOOK

In this workbook, you'll learn that what you eat determines whether your brain is in a responsive mode or a reactionary mode. Having protein along with carbohydrates in your meals and snacks optimizes your brain for energy and mental clarity, allowing anxiety, worry, and fatigue to drop away.

In chapter 1, the Snapshot of Anxiety Assessment helps identify the symptomatic details of your anxiety.

Chapter 2 guides you through a tool to help you learn the patterns of your anxiety. When does it show up? When is it better? Having these pieces in place will help you recognize the physiological patterns as they show up in your life.

Chapter 3 covers the physiology and addresses *why* protein is the solution.

In chapter 4, we give you the basic tools to reduce your anxiety within twenty minutes, lower your overall anxiety, and improve your energy over a three-day period. Although we do this with food, please understand that this is not a food program that you do now and forever. We provide a set of tools to be used as you move through your life. Some days you might use the tools throughout the day because you did the experiment and it helped so much that it's worth the effort, and some days you might not use the tools at all. But once you understand what helps in different situations, you can return to them when you're particularly challenged or are just tired of the chaos that life sometimes brings.

Chapter 5 teaches you how to read labels so you can predict how you'll feel after eating.

Chapter 6 explains how to plan your food so you feel like you can consistently manage your anxiety and reduce your fatigue.

Chapter 7 is about sleep, how it helps lower anxiety and fatigue, and techniques to reduce the anxiety symptoms that are associated with sleep.

Chapter 8 is about moving your body to protect your body's power supply. Even a small movement program supports the brain and body. We provide tools that improve energy and reduce anxiety in the moment, in as little as thirty seconds!

Chapter 9 is about how to work with your primary care provider if these solutions aren't enough.

In the appendix, you will find instructions and worksheets for the tools presented in each chapter. If you want, you can jump ahead and follow the instructions; if you need to know why the tools work, explanations are provided in the associated chapters.

A few more things to keep in mind: This book is educational; it should not be used as a replacement for professional health care providers. If you're working with a prescriber or therapist, please share with them what you're learning. If you're on medications for mental health or physical health, be sure to share any changes you make or are thinking of making with your physicians. If your conditions are complex, perhaps working through this book with a provider will be useful. Also note that this book is directed at individuals who are responsible for their own lives (likely sixteen years old and up). The information can be applied to younger individuals, but they would need to work with a caring, curious, and supportive adult.

Our ultimate goal is for you to have more energy and mental clarity, and more hope for what is possible in your life. More than a decade ago Dr. Chan Hellman set out to understand how hope impacts individuals in what appear to be hopeless situations. He discovered that people who have hope can successfully emerge out of enormous personal challenges. In the book *HOPE Rising*, Hellman and his colleague Casey Gwinn (2019) define hope as "the belief that a thriving future is possible, and you have the power to make it so" (31). Gwinn and Hellman build on researcher Rick

Snyder's work by identifying two key components of hope: willpower, what excites you and is unique to you and your motivations along with the power supply to follow through on changes you resolve to make, and "waypower," the ability to overcome challenges and the emotions that come with challenges.

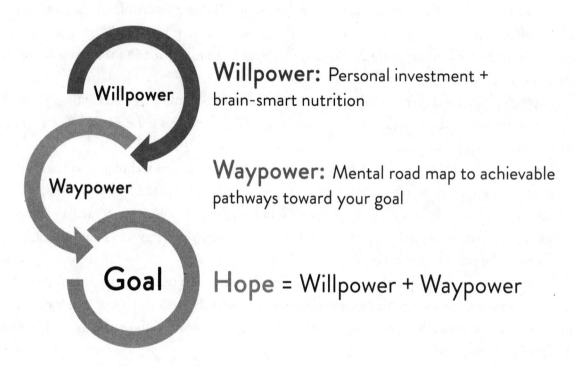

Willpower: Personal investment + brain-smart nutrition

Waypower: Mental road map to achievable pathways toward your goal

Hope = Willpower + Waypower

Hope is the belief that a thriving future is possible and you have the power to make it so.

We think this work is significant because many people have lost hope for achieving their dreams because their anxiety, worry, and fatigue have sapped them of the energy and mental clarity needed to stay in their responsive-cortex brains. And we have found that when people don't have the knowledge and tools to consistently maintain their bodies' power supply, which is the basis of willpower, it's difficult if not impossible to actually achieve their goals. This workbook provides tools for increasing both willpower and waypower; we want you to have the hope that a thriving future is possible and the tools needed to achieve it.

Let's start with the Snapshot of Anxiety Assessment in chapter 1 to understand all the symptoms of your anxiety, worry, and fatigue. The first step to reducing your symptoms is to assess which are specific to you.

Part I

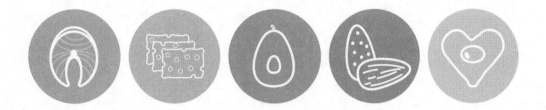

The Fundamentals of Glucose Regulation as a Solution for Anxiety and Fatigue

## CHAPTER 1

Snapshot of Anxiety

The Snapshot of Anxiety Assessment helps provide a clear picture of both the physical symptoms of anxiety and the other associated problems that accompany it. Not everyone experiences anxiety in the same way. Understanding what your anxiety looks like and the other symptoms that coexist with it, such as worry and fatigue, is the first step in improving your symptoms so you can more fully engage in your life.

The Snapshot of Anxiety Assessment is a questionnaire that helps you accurately characterize your anxiety. It has three sections that identify categories of the most common symptoms that coexist with anxiety. The purpose of doing the assessment is to better observe what your anxiety looks like and to begin to get a sense of what symptoms may be originating from physiological causes. In future chapters, we'll offer experiments to lower some of the symptoms of anxiety; getting this baseline up front will help you track your symptoms and identify which experiments will have the most positive impact.

PART 1: YOUR FATIGUE SCORE

The power supply from your body can determine your energy, mental clarity, and level of anxiety. Take a moment to rate your power supply—or how much energy you feel you have—on a scale of 1 to 10, with 1 being minimal energy and 10 being solid energy throughout the day. This isn't uncontrolled manic energy; a rating of 10 means that you have the resources to respond to whatever opportunities arise, good or challenging.

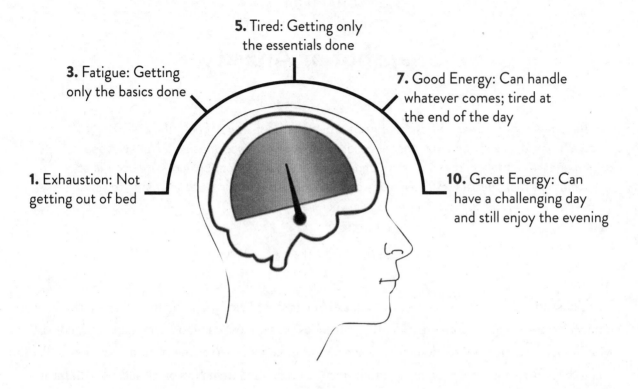

5. Tired: Getting only the essentials done

3. Fatigue: Getting only the basics done

7. Good Energy: Can handle whatever comes; tired at the end of the day

1. Exhaustion: Not getting out of bed

10. Great Energy: Can have a challenging day and still enjoy the evening

What is your power supply right now? _____

In general, what was your power supply like over the last two weeks? _____

What was your high? _____

What was your low? _____

If your energy is routinely dropping below a 5, that's not good. You may not have the energy to engage in novelty, you're possibly withdrawing from relationships, and the fatigue creates a physical reason to be anxious. When you're living at a 5 or below, it's hard to move your life forward, and it's hard to have hope for your future. The experiments in this book will help, both in the short and in the long term. And if they don't help enough, the last chapter provides some information about talking to your primary care provider about fatigue.

If your power supply drops below 5 during the active part of your day, give yourself a fatigue score of 10 points. If your power supply stays above 5, your fatigue score is 0.

Fatigue score: _____

PART 2: BRAIN–BODY SYMPTOMS

Below are the different brain and body symptoms of anxiety. If *any part* of a particular symptom description fits you, check the box and circle the part you relate to. Feel free to add other symptoms that are consistent with your anxiety but aren't listed or add qualifiers to the symptoms that are listed. There are 22 brain–body symptoms listed below; after going through the symptoms, add up the number of boxes that you checked, giving yourself one point per box to determine your total.

Brain Symptoms

☐ Flight emotions: agitation, nervousness, worry, anxiety, fear, panic

☐ Fight emotions: hyperfocused, defensive, negative, irritable, controlling, enraged

☐ Disappear emotions: withdrawn, depressed, crying, shut down

☐ Racing thoughts

☐ Negative thought patterns toward self, self-critical

☐ Emotional outbursts that are larger than necessary

☐ Doing old behaviors that you don't want to do again, such as eating sugar, drinking alcohol or using other addictive substances, or calling people who are not helpful

☐ Fear of dying, suicidal thoughts, confusion, abnormal behavior—*If you check this box, please ask for help, call a friend, call 911 or the crisis line in your area, or seek out a therapist.*

> ### Common "Disappear" Behaviors
>
> - Spending hours on the internet or social media (not work-related)
> - Overeating/undereating
> - Drinking alone or to excess
> - Using drugs alone or to excess
> - Watching TV for many hours
>
> *To identify a disappear behavior, ask yourself if you think an activity is a form of withdrawing or shutting down.*

Body Symptoms

- ☐ Shaky or trembling hands

- ☐ Heart palpitations, racing heart rate

- ☐ Shortness of breath

- ☐ Pale skin, cold hands or feet

- ☐ Shakiness, vibrating body, physically agitated, or fidgety

- ☐ Hungry, craving sugar, sweets, or carbohydrates (breads, pasta, candy)

- ☐ Nausea

- ☐ Not hungry for meals or not able to eat

- ☐ Sweating

- ☐ Dizziness

- ☐ Vertigo

- ☐ Visual disturbance

- ☐ Extreme fatigue

- ☐ Seizures or loss of consciousness

Brain and body symptoms score: _____

PART 3: GLOBAL SYMPTOMS

Global symptoms develop as the body copes with stress hormones over the long term. These symptoms both cause anxiety and are caused by anxiety. Use the rating scale provided to answer the global symptoms questions; skip questions that don't apply to you. Then, add the totals from each column to get your score.

Please rate these symptoms	Not at all	Some days	Most days	Nearly every day
Fatigue	0	1	2	3
Afternoon fatigue	0	1	2	3
Moodiness, including emotions of anxiety, irritation, agitation, and sadness	0	1	2	3
Lack of mental clarity	0	1	2	3
Morning insomnia/waking too early	0	1	2	3
Inability to wake up in morning	0	1	2	3
PTSD nightmares	0	1	2	3
Brain fog/harder to think	0	1	2	3
Physical pain for any cause	0	1	2	3
Distraction and/or ADHD symptoms	0	1	2	3
Dysregulated bowel symptoms (constipation, diarrhea, bloating)	0	1	2	3
Sugar/carbohydrate cravings	0	1	2	3
The use of alcohol or other substances to regulate your emotions and symptoms	0	1	2	3
Subtotals:				
Global symptoms score (add the scores from the four columns above):				

PART 4: SNAPSHOT OF ANXIETY SCORE

Write in the totals from parts 1, 2, and 3 to get your Snapshot of Anxiety score:

	Points
From Part 1: Fatigue score	
From Part 2: Brain and body symptoms score	
From Part 3: Global symptoms score	
Snapshot of Anxiety score (total from parts 1, 2, and 3):	

You might be curious about how to interpret your final score. However, when it comes to the Snapshot of Anxiety, there isn't a standard total. Instead, you'll be using the score to see if your ratings for each category and your total improve when you do experiments.

Once you've completed your snapshot, take a moment to reflect on any insights that you have gained.

You might have written about how many symptoms of anxiety and fatigue you're currently experiencing and the things in your life that are hard to do because of these symptoms. Considering the problems anxiety, worry, and fatigue cause can be helpful in motivating you to change. What can also be motivating—and is often even more motivating than fixing a problem—is pursuing the benefits that lower levels of anxiety, worry, and fatigue might give you. Let's consider some of these benefits now.

THE BENEFITS OF LOWER ANXIETY

Below are some benefits you may experience from reducing anxiety and having more time and energy to engage in your life. Use the table to rate their importance and add any other benefits that you're willing to actively work toward.

Benefits	Not important	Somewhat important	Mostly important	Very important
Feel better				
Better sleep				
More confident				
More at ease with yourself				
Willing to try new things				
Better connections and/or boundaries with friends and family				
Better able to take care of important projects				
Other:				

CHAPTER SUMMARY

By using the Snapshot of Anxiety Assessment, you can see that your anxiety has both symptoms that reside in your brain and symptoms that reside in your body. Every person's anxiety is somewhat different. Identifying what yours looks like is helpful for a number of reasons. First, the experiments in the coming chapters will help you reduce symptoms of fatigue, brain–body symptoms, and global symptoms. If you have less fatigue, racing thoughts, and sugar cravings, you'll find it easier to feel less anxious. This chapter also helped you identify the benefits of reducing anxiety. As you go through the workbook and learn new tools, we'll encourage you to return to the Snapshot of Anxiety Assessment to see which tool reduced which symptoms. Lastly, sometimes it's helpful to have a specific list of symptoms to describe what is happening if you're working with a therapist or primary care provider. The Snapshot of Anxiety Assessment worksheet is available in the appendix and for download at http://www.newharbinger.com/46233.

In the next chapter, you'll work on discovering *when* you're feeling anxious, what might be making you feel worse, and what might help you feel better.

## CHAPTER 2

What Impacts Anxiety

Understanding what impacts anxiety and recognizing patterns of how the symptoms of anxiety show up in your life gives you a starting place for using food, sleep, exercise, and other tools to improve anxiety, worry, and fatigue.

Food, sleep, and exercise determine your body's power supply. This means they can be significant drivers in your anxiety and fatigue; it also means they can be significant factors to reduce that anxiety and fatigue. The What Impacts Anxiety worksheet provides you with:

- A tool to increase awareness of the patterns of your anxiety. By identifying our patterns, we can often take action on our own behalf to address them before our anxiety accelerates and feels out of control.

- A reference point against which to measure the effect of experiments suggested in this workbook or other interventions, such as mindfulness, exposure therapy, medications, and observing anxiety levels in different environments or around different people.

- Documentation to share with medical care providers, if you're seeing any, to help you get better care in the limited time you have with them.

You don't have to use this tool as it's presented; you can use the information outlined to ask yourself what is responsible for accelerating or calming your anxiety on any given day.

THE WHAT IMPACTS ANXIETY WORKSHEET

Do you know what impacts your anxiety? The What Impacts Anxiety worksheet (also provided in the appendix and online at http://www.newharbinger.com/46233) will help you get more clear about this. We'll go through each component and explain how it may be affecting your anxiety, worry, and fatigue.

What Impacts Anxiety	Day 1 Date:	Day 2 Date:	Day 3 Date:
	What's going on?	What's going on?	What's going on?
Time of day			
Power Supply (1-10)			
ANXIETY LEVEL HIGH 10 9 8 7 / MED 6 5 4 / LOW 3 2 1			
Anxiety Accelerators (Caffeine, Alcohol, Sugary Foods, Screen Time, Stressful Day)			
Daily Practices:			
What did you eat (meal or snack)? (Protein, Carb, Veggie/Fiber, Fat)			
☑ Movement/Physical Activity			
☑ Safe, Supportive Connections			
Resiliency Factors (Mindfulness, Quiet Time, Time Outside, Spiritual Practice, Journaling)			
# of hours of sleep the night before			
Other Notes			

Brain diagram labels: 1. Fine, 3. Low, 5. Medium, 7. High, 10. Panic Attack/Total Shutdown

What's Going On?

Track what's going on as often as makes sense for you; you don't have to use all five columns provided. Examples might include meeting with your boss or client, transitioning from work to home, a phone call with a friend, or a tough conversation with a family member. The notes can be fairly basic; you can also use the back of the page if you need more space. The idea is to increase your awareness of what's going on throughout the day—both the highs and the lows—so you can begin to see your patterns and how these may be influenced by both accelerators and resilience factors.

What Impacts Anxiety	Day 1	Date:				Day 2	Date:				Day 3	Date:			
	What's going on?					What's going on?					What's going on?				
Time of day															
Power Supply (1-10)															

Time of Day

Note the time of day that corresponds to what you entered for "What's going on?"

Power Supply

It's important to check in regularly on your power supply, as this is what's helping your brain and mind stay calm and focused. Use the same scale from the power supply exercise in chapter 1: a scale of 1 to 10, with 1 being minimal energy and 10 being solid energy. Remember, a rating of 10 isn't uncontrolled manic energy; rather, it means that you have the resources to respond to whatever opportunity arises, good or challenging.

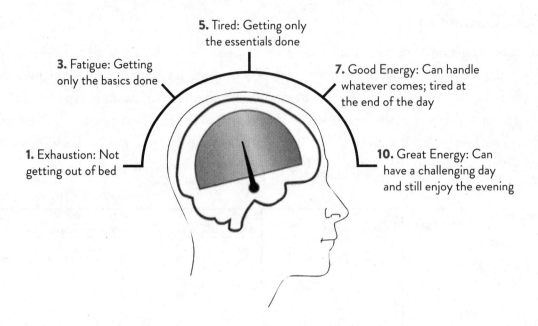

Anxiety Level

In this section, note the level of anxiety you felt, using the scale provided. Is it low, medium, high? Identifying what is low, medium, and high anxiety is unique to each individual. Remember the symptoms you identified in the Snapshot of Anxiety Assessment: What symptoms show up first? What symptoms show up only when anxiety is really high? These may change over time or in different situations.

One challenge with anxiety is that generally, we observe it when it's high and bothering us and we are uncomfortable; when it's not high, we may not think about anxiety at all. Another challenge is anxiety's lasting or residual effects. If we felt anxious at several points throughout the day, the different experiences aggregate in our memory, so the whole day gets labeled as anxious. This is why it's important to note when you're feeling anxious—so you can say, "I was anxious at lunchtime," and the whole day doesn't get colored as anxious. Fundamentally, the point of the exercise is to recognize that anxiety levels change throughout the day and week and to stay curious about what makes you feel better or worse.

For some people it can take some practice to learn to observe anxiety and to be able to determine its level. If the 1-to-10 scale is too difficult to identify with, you can just use the labels low (managing anxiety with little effort), medium (needing to start using tools to manage anxiety), and high (feeling really uncomfortable). As Dan Siegel (2010) says, you have to "name it to tame it."

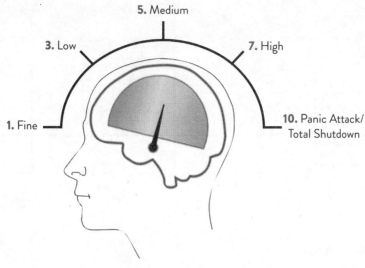

What is your anxiety level?

- *Low anxiety (levels 1–3)* is when you're mostly comfortable and are managing your anxiety with little effort. As you move from level 1 up to 3, you may be increasingly aware of it, but are still in control of how you're managing yourself.

- *Medium anxiety (levels 4–6)* is when you feel more uncomfortable and the symptoms of anxiety are drawing your attention and may begin impacting the decisions and actions you take. This is when you need to start pulling out your tools to manage the anxiety. This worksheet helps you identify your triggers and when you need to be thinking about using those tools. It's normal to have medium levels of anxiety off and on through life, such as when doing something new, before a presentation, or when returning to something that was really hard.

- *High anxiety (levels 7–10)* is when you start feeling really uncomfortable. This is where decision making and behavior are starting to be heavily influenced by the anxiety. The anxiety may no longer feel manageable, or you may feel like you're just holding on. Left unchecked, you may experience a panic attack or total shutdown.

Although you may be curious as to how your anxiety level compares with others', this worksheet is intended to help *you* characterize *your* sense of it. Any comparison is to yourself, over time, and with experiments that you do to manage your anxiety better.

ANXIETY LEVEL	HIGH	10														
		9														
		8														
		7														
	MED	6														
		5														
		4														
	LOW	3														
		2														
		1														
Anxiety Accelerators (Caffeine, Alcohol, Sugary Foods, Screen Time, Stressful Day)																

Anxiety Accelerators

Some things accelerate anxiety. Keeping track of your accelerators, especially alongside your anxiety levels across different times of day, can help you identify what is driving your patterns of anxiety. Accelerators include:

- *Caffeine.* You may have fatigue and need caffeine to function, but caffeine makes it easier for your brain to be anxious and harder to sleep. Caffeine helps you feel awake by increasing the hypervigilance of your brain. Hypervigilance is a key symptom of some forms of anxiety. If you're prone to panic attacks, increasing the amount of information your brain is taking in might not be helpful. Stopping caffeine can keep anxiety from accelerating.

> ### Caffeine
>
> In general we try not to take beloved foods away from people, so if you're consuming more than two servings of caffeine a day and you really don't want to give it up altogether, first do the experiments in this book and see if your fatigue and anxiety get better through other interventions.

- *Alcohol.* Some people notice that, in the short term, a glass of alcohol helps reduce their anxiety. However, because alcohol disrupts your brain's fuel supply, you can start to experience symptoms of anxiety four to six hours later. The use of alcohol to calm anxiety in the evening can cause early-morning insomnia, nightmares, higher anxiety levels in the mornings, and may also contribute to anxiety throughout the day (Lydon et al. 2016).

- *Sugary foods.* Your brain begins to think that everything will be okay 20 to 60 minutes after consuming sugar, thanks to the quick hit of glucose. However, if the sugar isn't paired with protein, good fat, and healthy fiber, your blood glucose rapidly drops, and your anxiety starts to climb again within one and a half to three hours. We will discuss this phenomenon in more detail in chapter 3.

- *Screen time.* Spending more than two hours a day in front of a screen outside of work or school will increase anxiety, depression, and fatigue (Hoare et al. 2017; Madhav et al. 2017).

- *Stressful day.* We all understand how stress increases anxiety: as the things that trigger your anxiety pile up—long work hours, meetings, appointments, childcare—the symptoms you feel become worse and worse. During these busy days, your brain will need more fuel to manage the stress, your anxiety, and sugar cravings.

Daily Practices

Daily Practices:												
What did you eat (meal or snack)? (Protein, Carb, Veggie/Fiber, Fat)												
☑ **Movement/Physical Activity**												
☑ **Safe, Supportive Connections**												
Resiliency Factors (Mindfulness, Quiet Time, Time Outside, Spiritual Practice, Journaling)												
# of hours of sleep the night before												
Other Notes												

What and when you eat, movement and exercise, sleep, and supportive relationships are all important for maintaining your power supply and reducing anxiety. Conversely, not eating or eating foods without protein, not moving or exercising, not getting at least seven hours of sleep, and having to deal with unsupportive relationships can make managing anxiety more challenging. For your daily practices, just note what you're currently doing or not doing, without judgment. Do you notice any patterns that relate to your anxiety levels? We'll go into more detail about what might be driving these patterns in later chapters and will suggest achievable experiments for you to try, which may improve your anxiety, worry, and fatigue.

"Resilience factors" are additional things that help reduce anxiety. Keeping track of your resilience factors, especially alongside your anxiety levels across different times of day, can help you identify what may reduce your anxiety. In the worksheet, we've listed some common resilience factors. Maybe you have tried these or others. There are entire books written on each of these if you want to learn more.

Now that you know how the What Impacts Anxiety worksheet works, it's time to begin using it. When is a good day for you to start tracking the accelerators and resilience factors of your anxiety? Start on a day that might cause moderate anxiety, instead of a day that you anticipate will be extra challenging. This way, you won't be adding an additional task on an overwhelming day. We suggest using the worksheet to track your anxiety for three days.

A Visit with Extended Family

A few weeks ago Taylor spent a long weekend with family. Having worked with Kristen for some time now, she loaded up on protein snacks and protein-based ingredients for meals. Anticipating that this would likely be a stressful weekend, she decided to bring along the What Impacts Anxiety worksheet and give it a try.

Taylor started off thinking she would check in five times throughout the day, at regular intervals, but it quickly became clear that wasn't realistic given the setting. Still, she found that having started with this intention kept her checking in with herself much more regularly than she would have otherwise. Taylor generally jotted notes on the worksheet at the beginning and end of each day, noting the ups and downs as she remembered them.

What Impacts Anxiety

Anxiety Level scale (head diagram): 10. Panic Attack/Total Shutdown · 7. High · 5. Medium · 3. Low · 1. Fine

ANXIETY LEVEL — Power Supply (1–10): HIGH (10, 9, 8), MED (7, 6, 5, 4), LOW (3, 2, 1)

Day 1 — Date: Sat 6/24 — What's going on?

Category	Woke up (6:30a)	Family outing (10a)	Errands on my own (12p)	Family meeting (4p)	~1 hour after dinner (9p)
Power Supply (1–10)	8	7	7	7	6
Anxiety Level (X)	2	8	4	8	5
Anxiety Accelerators	C	C	SF		A, SD
What did you eat (meal or snack)?	P, V, F	P, C	P		P
☑ Movement/Physical Activity		✓	✓		✓
☑ Safe, Supportive Connections					
Resiliency Factors			O	M	J
# hours of sleep night before	~8				
Other Notes	P w/meals/snacks throughout day				

Day 2 — Date: Sun 6/25 — What's going on?

Category	Woke up (6a)	Family conversation (8a)	Preparing lunch (12p)	~1 hour after dinner (8p)	Late night conversation (11p)
Power Supply (1–10)	8	6	7	7	5
Anxiety Level (X)	3	6	4	4	6
Anxiety Accelerators	C	C		SF	A, SD
What did you eat (meal or snack)?	P, C, F		P, C, V, F		P
☑ Movement/Physical Activity			✓		
☑ Safe, Supportive Connections			✓		
Resiliency Factors	Q			O	J
# hours of sleep night before	~9, but interrupted				
Other Notes	P throughout day				

Day 3 — Date: Mon 6/26 — What's going on?

Category	Prepared to leave (7:30a)	Did not leave on time (8:30a)	Arrived home (2p)	~2 hours after dinner (8:30p)
Power Supply (1–10)	5	7	6	8
Anxiety Level (X)	4	7	6	8
Anxiety Accelerators	C			SD
What did you eat (meal or snack)?	P, C, F		P, C	P
☑ Movement/Physical Activity				✓
☑ Safe, Supportive Connections				
Resiliency Factors	Q			J
# hours of sleep night before	~7, interrupted			
Other Notes	1st time no panic attack at in-laws			

Anxiety Accelerators (Caffeine, Alcohol, Sugary Foods, Screen Time, Stressful Day)

Daily Practices throughout the day:

What did you eat (meal or snack)? (Protein, Carb, Veggie/Fiber, Fat)

Resiliency Factors (Mindfulness, Quiet Time, Time Outside, Spiritual Practice, Journaling)

Being more aware helped her to know when to pull out her "tools," like taking a quick time-out or grabbing some beef jerky or a hard-boiled egg. She also made a point of going to bed at her normal time (ten to eleven o'clock), even though everyone else was staying up until 2:00 or 3:00 a.m. Taylor realized on the first morning that this had an added benefit of some quiet time, as she also woke up a bit earlier than everyone else.

Although there were a few acute stress points throughout the weekend, Taylor's anxiety over the weekend was lower than during previous visits. As she drove home, she realized that she didn't need a day off from work to recover the way she did after previous family gatherings.

CHAPTER SUMMARY

Hopefully, after you've used the What Impacts Anxiety worksheet for a brief period of time, you now have a better sense of what's influencing your anxiety. The What Impacts Anxiety worksheet is available in the appendix and for download at http://www.newharbinger.com/46233.

Next we'll explain why the food you eat is such an important factor in your experience of anxiety, as an accelerator *and* a resilience factor. Armed with this knowledge, you'll be able to begin using food as a tool to manage anxiety.

## CHAPTER 3

A Fueled Brain Is a Less Anxious Brain

Instead of addressing food in terms of calories or fat content, we look at dietary choices from the perspective of how food will make you feel today and tomorrow. To help you have this insight, we explain how the brain and body function to escalate or reduce your anxiety and fatigue. We'll review the parts of the brain and the hormones that contribute either to anxiety or to helping you be at your best.

Understanding *why* you might be anxious or fatigued is important to improving how you feel. This chapter introduces the physiology that contributes to or improves anxiety, worry, and fatigue. The physiology you will be learning about is directly related to a host of conditions in which anxiety might be a factor:

- General anxiety and panic attacks

- Specific anxiety: phobias, performance anxiety, social anxiety, obsessive-compulsive disorder, and anxiety around high-stakes decision making

- Early-morning waking, waking with anxiety or irritation, or not being able to wake up in the morning

- Symptoms of post-traumatic stress disorder (PTSD), including nightmares and night terrors

- Sugar cravings

- Fatigue in general, and afternoon fatigue specifically

We'll be talking about solutions for all of these in the coming chapters. For those of you thinking, *I'm not a science person*, rest assured that we have explained the concepts in this chapter to thousands of people who don't have a science background. They appreciated having the physiology explained in accessible terms because it helped them understand why they were experiencing anxiety, worry, and fatigue. We also provide a story about a woman named Luca. You'll see this physiology play out through her story and will likely recognize in yourself some of what is happening to her.

The reality is that some food choices either contribute to anxiety—as well as worry, irritation, agitation, sugar cravings, and fatigue—or improve energy, mental clarity, and decision making. To understand this connection, you need to understand *glucose regulation—the process by which glucose levels are maintained in your bloodstream*. This explains the *why*; later in the workbook we'll cover the what, how, and when.

Your power supply for your body and your brain is determined in part by the types of food you consume. We're going to examine dietary choices from the perspective of brain optimization through glucose regulation. When we don't provide our bodies with the foods they need to fuel our brains, energy and mental clarity can go down the drain; chaotic days can become horrible days, causing fatigue, anxiety, irritability, and sugar cravings…to name but a few unsavory effects.

Our goal is to give you an understanding of how your food choices can help your body remain energetic and your mind clear. When we truly understand our bodies and their physiological processes, we can better observe, assess, and change what we experience. We can make better choices and navigate our chaotic lives with newfound grace and resilience. Anxiety can become more manageable even on emotionally challenging days, and the post-challenge fatigue will recede faster. We'll start by exploring a potentially familiar storyline.

Luca's Anxiety and Fatigue Get in the Way of a Promotion

Luca is the mother of two children. Before work, she prepares breakfast for her kids, feeds the dog, and readies everyone to leave the house. She makes a cup of coffee to drink in the car at 7:30 a.m. On a good day, she finishes the cereal that the kids didn't eat for breakfast. Otherwise, she grabs a piece of toast on her way out the door. For lunch, she often eats either a Caesar salad with low-fat dressing or spaghetti with red sauce. She strives to choose salad because she thinks it's the best choice. Her doctor says that her "good" cholesterol is too low. Her efforts to lose weight are challenged by the office secretary who keeps a bottomless bowl of candy at her desk and encourages people to help themselves. That said, the workplace also aids Luca's health endeavors: Luca and her colleague Raz walk together for thirty minutes during their lunch break.

Luca's hoping to be hired for a different position within her company. However, in the role that she desires, she would have to engage in more public speaking and assume more significant leadership. In her current position, she's very effective and confident with her work, and she's comfortable working with people one-on-one. The responsibilities of the new position would expand well beyond her current projects. Luca's not sure if she would be able to control the resulting anxiety that she is already anticipating. In the past, public speaking has been a disaster for Luca. Her brain races with those failures and tells her she is too stupid to successfully do the presentations, even though all evidence is to the contrary. The last time she had to give a presentation, her hands were shaking, and she felt like she was going to pass out because her heart was racing so fast. Before the event, she was so nauseated that she couldn't eat breakfast. Everyone said she did fine, and her boss encouraged her to apply for the job because her analysis in the presentation was so useful to the project. But for Luca, there was nothing that felt "fine" about it. Part of her never wants to experience that again. Part of what comes up for Luca is her childhood. Her mother drank heavily and would yell at her when she asked for help with her homework, telling her that she was stupid; public presentation feels the same as when she needed help from her mother as a child.

After work, when Luca picks up her kids at 4:00 p.m., she's exhausted and more irritable with them than she would like. After arriving home and settling the children into an activity, she pours herself a glass of wine before making dinner. For dinner, she and her family usually eat chicken, a green vegetable, and some potato preparation (such as mashed or baked potatoes or French fries). The potato dishes are her fussy children's primary sources of vegetables.

Often, Luca drinks another glass of wine with her husband during dinner. Then at 8:00 p.m., the kids go to bed, which allows her enough time to clean the house, answer emails, talk with her husband, and watch some television. She typically goes to bed by 11:00 p.m. Increasingly, though, she's been waking up at 3:00 a.m. thinking about all the tasks on her to-do list. Around 5:00 a.m., she falls back asleep only to be awakened by her alarm at 6:00 a.m. She's fairly sure that this sleep–wake cycle is why she's exhausted by the afternoon.

Luca seems to be doing many things right: she usually eats breakfast and regularly has vegetables with dinner, and she exercises. But despite her efforts, she's exhausted. She feels that her anxiety is holding her back from advancement within her company. She's hungry throughout the day and can't stop herself from eating candy at work. She's irritable with her kids, and she's not sleeping through the night.

To understand what's happening with Luca, we must understand the physiology of the predicaments her body and brain are experiencing. You may intuitively recognize some of this, but maybe no one has explained the science to you. When you understand the why, it becomes easier to do the what and how and to know the when.

WHERE DOES ANXIETY COME FROM?

To understand why sometimes Luca feels anxious and sometimes she is calm and confident, we need to understand the brain. Different parts of the brain provide different emotional and behavioral responses to the sensory input we receive from the world around us.

The **cerebral cortex**, which consists of two large hemispheres situated beside each other near the front and top of the brain, is the part of the brain unique to humans. The cerebral cortex provides us with the capacity for self-awareness, connection to others, problem solving, memory, learning, and organization. It also requires a lot of energy in the form of glucose to do all this amazing human work (Sprague and Arbeláez 2011; Warren and Frier 2005). When Luca feels confident and successful, her cerebral cortex is mainly in charge of thinking and emotions. When she is in this part of her brain, she feels like herself.

The **hippocampus** sits just below the cerebral cortex. It serves as Grand Central Station for almost all ingoing and outgoing information. Together, the hippocampus and the cerebral cortex help us assess and navigate our world, thereby fostering intentional, appropriate, and creative decision making and behavior.

The **limbic system** is the oldest part of our brain and the home base of our primitive and so-called lizard brain. The limbic system is involved in the following instinctual reactions: *fight, flight, disappear,* and *default to the old habit.* Some people classify these instincts as *flight, fight,* and *freeze.* However, considering typical human behavior, *disappear* seems more accurate than freeze. For example, we disappear out of our conscious thoughts into potato chips, ice cream, social media, or alcohol. The other programming that the limbic system is in charge of is defaulting to an old habit or behavior. Much of what we do relies on habitual behaviors or past behaviors. Some of those habitual behaviors may have helped us survive in the past, but they're not always useful when we have to navigate present circumstances creatively.

Traumas from childhood can trigger default reactions. For Luca, being raised by a single mom who was often drunk was stressful as a child, particularly on nights when she needed help with her homework. Even though Luca is no longer a child, and a work presentation isn't schoolwork, these are linked at a deeper level in Luca's brain and body. The limbic system pulls up the associated emotions and behaviors, such as her mother's rant, "You're so stupid," which isn't a useful phrase to hear for anyone at any time. Even though Luca is now an adult, successfully navigating a job, her lizard brain defaults to the old memories when she's doing something new, escalating her anxiety.

All three sections of the brain—the **cerebral cortex**, **hippocampus**, and **limbic system**—are used differently depending on circumstance and how we have fueled our bodies. When we feel safe, relaxed, and well fed, the input derived from sensing our world travels to higher-functioning parts of the brain: the *cerebral cortex* and the *hippocampus*. (We refer to these parts of the brain as the "responsive-cortex brain.") These parts of the brain enable us to make clear and sound decisions, even amid complex situations and problems. When you're in your responsive-cortex brain, you're conscious, able to learn, and able to make appropriate and creative decisions based on both past experiences and present information.

By contrast, when we feel unsafe, stressed, or underfed, adrenaline is released. Our bodies release adrenaline during trials, such as during crises at work or school, when our children are unsafe, or when our brains are running low on glucose. Adrenaline engages our *reactive-limbic system*. When the brain is exposed to adrenaline, sensory input stops traveling primarily to the cerebral cortex and hippocampus (the smart, responsive-cortex brain) and is instead routed to the reactive-limbic system. Once the reactive-limbic part of the brain becomes the primary recipient of sensory input, it's forced to choose from the four instinctual reactions: *fight, flight, disappear,* or *default to a habit from the past.*

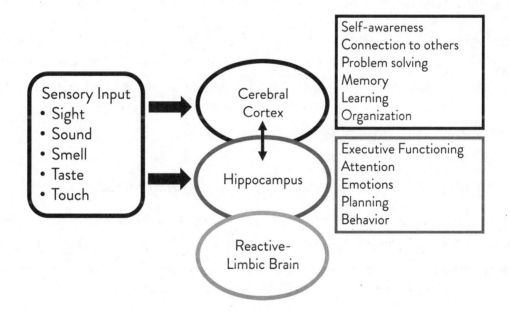

The smart, responsive-cortex brain is made up of the cerebral cortex and hippocampus. When your brain is well fueled, sensory input is interpreted by the smart, responsive-cortex brain, and you can make clear and sound decisions, even amid complex situations and problems, and are more oriented to the present moment and future.

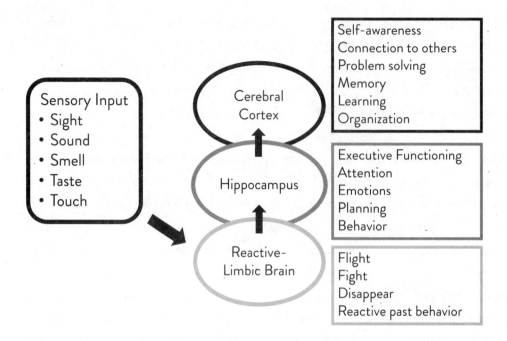

When not well fueled, sensory input is interpreted first from the reactive-limbic brain. We then react habitually, driven by negative emotions, like anxiety, irritation, or numbness; the responsive-cortex brain rides in the backseat.

This is why the unsupportive words from Luca's mother return when Luca gets anxious with something new or hard or if she simply has not eaten in a long time. The problem with adrenaline being released because of an internal physiological problem, such as low blood sugar, is that it's hard to identify the cause. If we get anxious because a bear walked into the room, we're pretty clear why our body is creating the sensations of anxiety.

UNDERSTANDING THE REACTIVE-LIMBIC SYSTEM

When the lizard brain is in charge, we end up in our *reactive-limbic brain:* reacting habitually, driven by negative emotions, like anxiety, irritation, or numbness. The responsive-cortex brain rides in the backseat. Sometimes backseat drivers are heard, and at other times they're not. Under these conditions, people experience one or more of the following:

Fight

- Irritation

- Agitation

- Anger

- Rage

Disappear (or Freeze)

- Mindless consumption of foods such as potato chips and ice cream

- Inability to focus or concentrate

- Being on autopilot

- Conservation of energy; feeling like you're moving in slow motion; sudden bouts of fatigue

- Helplessness

- Feeling trapped

- Numbness

- Disassociation; out-of-body experience

Flight

- Inattentiveness

- Scattered thoughts

- Nervousness

- Anxiety

- Panic attack

Default to a Habit from the Past

- Return to and reliance on past behaviors or habits that aren't presently most useful

- Denying the validity of new information despite present relevance

- PTSD flashbacks

This also applies to Luca. When she comes home and has not eaten in a while, her anxiety and irritation about her kids are more active. Her brain isn't fueled enough for her to be the engaged and supportive mom she wants to be.

To summarize, when we're anxious, the reactive-limbic brain is in charge; it's trying to ensure our survival. But we all want more than just survival; we want connection, creativity, resilience, to be forward thinking, and to be present for what is happening in our lives. For all this to happen, we need to operate from the responsive-cortex brain. The cortex needs a lot of fuel to process all that is happening around us. What and when we eat can determine which of the two parts of our brains we're responding with.

HOW DIFFERENT FOODS POWER THE BODY AND THE BRAIN

Let's begin by taking a closer look at the different types of food we can use as the power supply for our brains and bodies. There are many ways to categorize food, and of course, there are lots of different opinions on what the "right diet" is. We want to be clear that the focus of this book is for *you* to learn how food affects *your* anxiety and fatigue. Until your anxiety is manageable and you have a stable power supply from the body, it will be tough for you to do or change anything else.

There are four types of dietary fuels: (1) *the quick*, carbohydrates; (2) *the stable*, protein; (3) *the satisfying*, fats; and (4) *the structure*, fiber.

1. The Quick: Carbohydrates

Carbohydrates are molecules that are made up of sugars, starch, and cellulose. When we eat carbohydrates, the sugars are broken down in our digestive systems into individual units of glucose—aka blood sugar, the preferred fuel of the brain—that our bodies absorb and use. Once glucose enters the bloodstream, it's quickly transported to various cells, such as those in the brain and muscles. Excess glucose, meaning that which cannot be immediately used by cells as fuel for the body, is converted into adipose tissue (fat) for long-term storage.

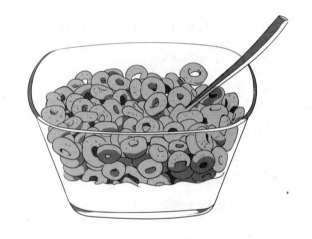

In modern life, carbohydrates are abundant and easy to get a hold of. This was not so true even two hundred years ago. The amount and frequency of our consumption of carbohydrates, without balancing them with protein, fat, and fiber, contribute to anxiety, fatigue, and other mental health problems (Firth et al. 2019; Jacka et al. 2010). Common foods that are mostly carbohydrates are breads, cereals, pasta, pastries, juice, candy, cookies, ice cream, and alcohol. Notice that most of these are manufactured foods. We can also count fruit, rice, and white potatoes as carbohydrates because they're converted quickly into glucose in the bloodstream. In this book, we don't include vegetables (tomatoes, carrots, bell peppers, lettuce, and spinach, to name a few) in this category, even though they're mostly made of cellulose, a carbohydrate, because they don't significantly affect your blood glucose.

In the end, when it comes to carbs, remember: it's not what you think of them that matters; it's how your body responds to them.

2. The Stable: Protein

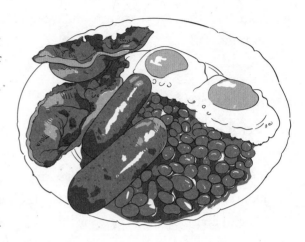

Protein is made up of amino acids, the building blocks of our bodies. Amino acids are the backbone of muscle, DNA, enzymes, ligaments, tendons, and neurotransmitters, such as dopamine and serotonin. Common sources of protein are meats (chicken, turkey, pork, beef); eggs (chicken, duck); fish (salmon, tuna, halibut); seafood (shrimp, scallops, mussels); legumes (beans, lentils); soy (tofu, tempeh, soy milk); protein powders (whey, soy, rice, pea); dairy from cows, sheep, and goats (yogurt, cottage cheese, milk, cheese); and nuts (almonds, cashews, hazelnuts, walnuts, peanuts).

When we consistently eat protein in our meals throughout the day, our glucose levels are more stable, reducing anxiety and improving fatigue. Protein can be converted into glucose by the liver if our brains and bodies are running low. This process is called "*gluconeogenesis*."

3. The Satisfying: Fat

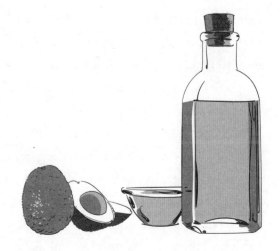

Fat can be both acquired directly from the diet and synthesized by the liver from carbohydrates or protein. Fats comprise the membranes of every cell in our bodies and make up the myelin sheaths that cover and protect our brain cells. Fat also helps protect our organs and is the backbone for the synthesis of important hormones. Thus, fat is essential for our bodies— so essential that if it's not in a meal, we don't get the physiological signal that the meal was satisfying. In other words, fat helps us stop feeling hungry.

For thirty years, the public health message was to avoid fats. Only recently has this messaging changed. During the "avoid fat" public health message campaign, milk and yogurts had fat partially or entirely removed, and we were taught to look for and choose "fat-free." What the processed-food industry didn't bother to say in the advertisements is that our bodies will happily take the sugar that's added into the fat-free yogurts and other products to make them palatable and convert the added sugar into fat!

4. The Structure: Fiber

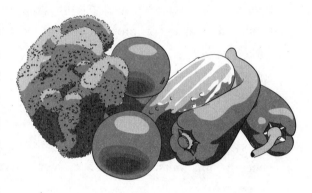

Fiber is technically a carbohydrate because it's made of cellulose. But because fiber is not absorbed into the bloodstream and stays in the digestive system, it doesn't become glucose. Thus, for this book, we're not going to consider fiber a carbohydrate. We are going to give it its own category. Fiber helps the digestive system work better by giving internal structure to what is otherwise a long tube. This structure does a lot of important things that support both physical and mental health. Fiber helps us have regular bowel movements. If you've ever gone three or four days without a bowel movement, you know that this can create anxiety and fatigue. It also helps remove fats, excess hormones, and waste products that the body no longer needs. When we eat low-fiber meals, we can end up reabsorbing stuff that we should be getting rid of. The "crap" that we reabsorb can increase our fatigue and decrease our mental clarity. Additionally, and for us most important, fiber helps us absorb nutrients. The brain requires a lot of vitamins and minerals. When we eat enough fiber, our digestive system works better and we're able to absorb what we need.

Let's look at two ways to include fiber in our diets: nutrient-rich fiber sources and fiber-rich foods. The best source of nutrient-rich fiber is vegetables! The fiber is like packaging that holds the vitamins, minerals, and other nutrients in place so that they can be released slowly enough to be absorbed into the bloodstream. Foods high in fiber and vitamins include artichokes, carrots, broccoli, Brussels sprouts, cabbage, lettuce, cucumbers, bell peppers, tomatoes, sweet potatoes, legumes (lentils, beans, peas, chickpeas), nuts, and whole grains that you cook (oats, quinoa, barley, millet). Like nutrient-rich foods, fiber-rich foods help our digestive system function better. Common sources of fiber-rich foods are the coarser parts of vegetables (stems, seeds, and skin), flaxseeds, chia seeds, and popcorn.

The latest science is showing that the bacteria in our digestive system can impact our mental health (Skonieczna-Żydecka et al., 2018). While the details of this are still being worked out, the take-home message is clear: doing what we can to support our digestive health will improve our energy and mental clarity.

KNOW YOUR SUPPLY CHAIN

It's important to know what the different fuel types are doing for your body.

- *Glucose* is the primary fuel for the brain, but more than that—all cells can use glucose as a fuel source. Glucose can also be converted into fat by the liver.

- *Protein* is the building block of the body and can be converted into glucose by the liver. Proteins help build every cell in our body, including cells in our brains.

- *Fat* forms the membranes of every cell in our body, is the backbone of many hormones, and helps us feel satisfied with a meal.

- *Fiber*-rich veggies provide essential vitamins, minerals, and nutrients for our brains and bodies. Fiber also helps our digestive system do its job of absorbing nutrients and removing wastes correctly.

Although the best combination in a meal is all four, getting them in all the time can be challenging. Getting enough protein with some carbohydrates is our focus for how to reduce anxiety, worry, and fatigue and improve how you feel in the moment so you can be at your best.

Now that you have a basic understanding of the four categories of foods that make up your meals and snacks, we want to introduce two hormones: insulin and adrenaline. These hormones contribute to anxiety because they influence your glucose levels, which fluctuate based on when and what you eat.

HOW FOODS IMPACT HORMONES AND HOW HORMONES DRIVE ANXIETY

Insulin is the hormone that encourages transport of glucose, amino acids, and fats into cells to be used either to build and maintain the cell or as fuel. The release of insulin from the pancreas is triggered any time we eat or drink something other than water. The amount of insulin released is dependent on several factors, including how much and how quickly glucose is entering the blood-stream from the digestive system. Highly processed high-carbohydrate foods that are low in fiber (candy, soda, juice, breads, cereals) cause the release of a lot of insulin compared to low-carbohydrate high-fiber foods, such as an apple or refried beans. When a large amount of insulin is released into the bloodstream, the nutrients from our food are quickly removed from circulation.

Adrenaline, also known as epinephrine, is a hormone released from the adrenal gland and some nerve cells. The purpose of adrenaline is to ensure that the body has the resources it needs to survive a stressful event. Adrenaline has several short- and long-term effects. For instance, adrenaline can increase your heart rate—and heart palpitations are one common symptom of anxiety. Adrenaline also moves blood to the muscles, away from skin (and true enough, pale skin and cold hands and feet can be a symptom or indicator of anxiety). Adrenaline also increases the rate of breathing (which explains why you can get short of breath when you're anxious), puts the body on full alert (explaining anxious shakiness, agitation, trembling, or fidgeting), increases the utilization of glucose in the brain (explaining the hunger or cravings for sugar or sweets that you can experience when you're anxious), increases sweating, and moves blood away from the digestive system, effectively slowing or stopping digestion so the body can focus on more immediate action (which explains why some people feel nausea or lack of appetite when they're anxious).

This chapter will help you recognize adrenaline and its effects in your life, as well as in other people's lives. Generally, adrenaline is released in moments of stress. It can also be released when the brain is running out of glucose. When this happens, the liver needs to convert protein into glucose (gluconeogenesis). While a host of other hormones is also used in this process, we're specifically tracking adrenaline because of its unique impact on the body and brain.

Adrenaline can create many of the symptoms we commonly label as anxiety, thus escalating physical symptoms of emotional distress. Luca may not even know that a hormone in her body makes her heart race, causes her hands to shake, and sends her thoughts racing. But there is one more sig-nificant problem for Luca and anyone who is plagued with anxiety: when adrenaline is in our blood-stream, all sensory input shifts from our smart, creative, connected, thoughtful responsive-cortex brain to our reactive-limbic system. Your reactive-limbic system perceives everything from the per-spective of fight (irritation), flight (anxiety), disappear (numbed-out behavior), or default habits or behaviors (responding from the past). In other words, when we're under stress *and* we haven't eaten or haven't eaten frequently enough, our bodies will produce even more adrenaline just to fuel our brains. This low-glucose, elevated-adrenaline physiology can cause many of the symptoms listed on the Snapshot of Anxiety Assessment. From Luca's story, her list of adrenaline-provoked experiences includes thinking about applying for a new job, doing presentations at work, and the transition from work to home life. Being without fuel makes these events worse.

If we have a history of trauma, we have extra receptors in our limbic system scanning for any adrenaline that might signal that we're in a survival situation. This means that we respond to smaller doses of adrenaline. If we know that this is happening, we can use our responsive-cortex brain to calm the response. In this book, we are focusing on how to reduce anxiety by understanding the importance of supplying our bodies and brains with the fuel needed to stay in the responsive-cortex brain so we can better manage our reactions and behavior. There are also therapeutic techniques and therapies that use the responsive-cortex brain to calm the reactive-limbic system: mindfulness, cognitive behavioral therapy, and dialectical behavioral therapy, to name a few.

THE ROLLER COASTER OF HORMONES CONTRIBUTING TO ANXIETY

Now, if we think back to Luca's story and look at it through the lens of insulin and adrenaline, we see in Luca's day a pattern that is common for many people: a breakfast dominated by carbohydrates and candy or refined carbohydrates throughout the day. The spike of insulin caused by eating refined carbs quickly depletes glucose in the bloodstream. As the brain and body detect a drop in glucose, hormones are released, including adrenaline, to stimulate the liver to create more glucose to replace what has been quickly used. As soon as the adrenaline reaches your brain, you switch from your responsive-cortex brain to your reactive-limbic brain. You now interpret the world through the filters of fight, flight, disappear, or play the old record from the past. The adrenaline is creating the physical symptoms of anxiety (racing heart, shortness of breath, nausea, lack of hunger) as well as impacting the brain by creating worry, anxiety, racing thoughts, and negative thought patterns. Let's look at this more closely.

Part 1: The Glucose-and-Insulin Roller Coaster

After we eat high-carbohydrate breakfasts (such as Luca's toast or cereal), our blood glucose and insulin levels surge. Insulin tells cells throughout the body that they should open their receptors to blood glucose, which then rushes into the cells to fuel and maintain them. It's crucial to understand that blood glucose levels are always in flux; blood glucose and insulin levels rapidly cycle through spikes and drops. More specifically, it takes about one and a half to two hours for insulin to clear the bloodstream following consumption of a carbohydrate-only meal or snack.

Part 2: Crashing: Here Comes the Anxiety

About one and half to two hours after a breakfast consisting mostly of carbohydrate (such as cereal, muffin, bagel, or toast), insulin has facilitated the cellular uptake of most of the blood glucose. This means that the glucose level in the bloodstream is dropping.

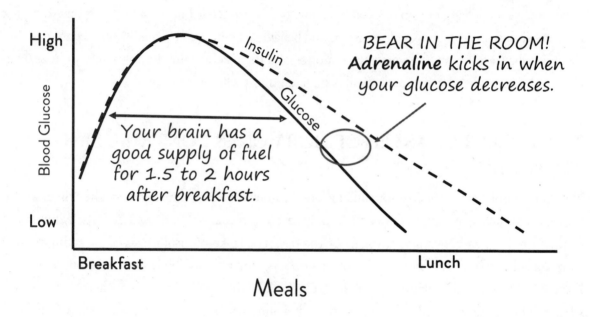

A Breakfast Without Protein

When the glucose level in the bloodstream drops, the brain begins to detect that its primary fuel source is getting low. Luca's brain might lament, "I need fuel to think. I have lots of work, loads and loads of email, text messages, and telephone calls to make. I wonder when I'll get some more sugar. Oh yeah, we won't. We just made a pledge to not eat from the office candy bowl, but some sugar would really help me think more clearly about the two hundred emails I need to respond to in the next hour…" Luca's brain is under the stress of trying to work without enough fuel.

Finally, her blood glucose levels drop so low that her brain hits the panic button and releases adrenaline into the bloodstream. The adrenaline release sets off a cascade of events that makes Luca operate from her reactive-limbic brain, typically resulting in increased anxiety symptoms. Under these conditions, she experiences emotional upset: irritability, overreacting to her kids, and anxiously limiting her career options.

Part 3: Short-Term Solution—Staying Fueled with Sugars

Many of us seem to put some kind of food into our bodies every two to three hours, not because we lack willpower but because our brains need fuel. Ironically, the sugar we often gravitate to in these moments moves us into our responsive-cortex brains, which is what gives us willpower. In other words, eating sugar is a physiologically smart short-term behavior: we're fueling our brains so we can stay in the responsive-cortex brain and keep the reactive-limbic system in the backseat. This is why Luca can't stop herself from eating a few pieces of candy each time she walks by the office secretary's bottomless bowl of bonbons. She craves the added boost that sweets temporarily supply. If she successfully resists these candies, her blood glucose levels will drop, and adrenaline will be released. This can cause anxiety symptoms during the day when nothing in particular is triggering them. This physiology is driven by her meal choices and contributes to her feeling anxious "all the time" and not feeling able to take on anything new. While consuming sugary or high-carbohydrate foods without other nutrients (protein, vegetables, high-fiber foods, healthy fats) is a short-term solution for getting through a busy day, over the long term, it can create both mental and physical health challenges.

I NEED HELP NOW!

A Lizard Brain Treat is a snack of sugar (a quick fuel) and protein (a longer-lasting fuel). You want the quick fuel to get to your brain almost immediately, which will start to reduce the adrenaline that's causing you to be in your reactive-limbic system (lizard brain). Including protein in the snack extends the amount of time you're in your responsive-cortex brain before needing to refuel. See the handout I Need Help Now! in the appendix for ideas for Lizard Brain Treats.

If any of the following are happening, try the Lizard Brain Treat experiment below.

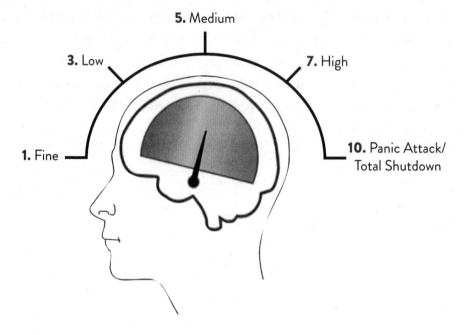

- Are you having a panic attack?

- Are you uncomfortably anxious or irritated?

- Are you overly or underly emotional for the situation?

- Do you want to feel better in 10 to 15 minutes?

Experiment

1. Circle your anxiety level before you have the Lizard Brain Treat.

2. Eat a quick fuel, like a quarter cup of juice, and a protein (a longer-lasting fuel), such as a handful of nuts or one of the ideas from the handout I Need Help Now! in the appendix.

3. Wait 10 to 15 minutes.

4. Check back in with yourself (after the 10 to 15 minutes) and rerate your anxiety level.

5. Are you feeling better? If your anxiety was due in part to low glucose and high adrenaline, your anxiety level has hopefully dropped by 10 to 30 percent, which likely feels better and allows you to use other tools to manage the anxiety, worry, or fatigue that may remain.

The "I Need Help Now!" handout is available in the appendix and for download at http://www .newharbinger.com/46233.

Part 4: Burnout: Long-Term Consequences of Adrenaline for the Body

The symptoms of anxiety happen one and a half to two hours after we eat refined carbohydrates without enough protein. After this time period, adrenaline signals for the liver to break down proteins into amino acids and convert them into glucose to replace the rapidly consumed carbohydrates. The protein comes from two possible sources: protein from our last meal (no more than three to four hours earlier) or from our muscle mass.

Let's take a moment to understand what our muscle mass has to do with anxiety. Our muscle mass sets our metabolic rates, which determine how many calories we can eat without contributing to our fat mass. If we steal little amounts of muscle by converting it into glucose for fuel day after day—which is what happens when we don't eat enough protein—we establish a pattern of adrenaline-related symptoms of anxiety. On top of this, we lower our muscle mass. Lower muscle mass makes it hard to have the physical strength to do the activities of our daily lives and contributes to fatigue. This sets us up to be anxious and fatigued all the time.

Ultimately, having low muscle mass—due to the combination of sedentary lifestyle, a low-protein diet, and using muscle as a fuel source—can cause people to become overweight. At this point, you might ask: Why do we bring up weight in an anxiety book? It's because mental and physical health are interrelated. It's vital to understand that the physiological processes we've been talking about contribute not only to your symptoms of anxiety and fatigue but also to weight gain and risk of diabetes. Also, for many people—though by no means for all people—weight is a contributor to emotional distress and anxiety as well as fatigue. Low muscle mass also increases the risk of developing type 2 diabetes, which is a glucose-regulation problem and can contribute to both anxiety and depression.

On the other hand, if we protect and build our muscle mass, by eating protein and carbohydrates regularly and moving our bodies more, then our muscles demand to be restocked—so more protein goes back into building our muscle mass and our glucose regulation is more stable. Protecting your muscle mass has been shown to help with anxiety, depression, the prevention of cognitive decline associated with aging, and a whole host of other physical health problems that we will discuss in the chapter on movement.

Another benefit from building muscle mass is that when we move our bodies, muscles release brain-derived neurotrophic factor (BDNF). BDNF is a compound called a neuropeptide, which acts as fertilizer for the brain: it helps us learn faster, encode memories, and do higher-level thinking. It helps the nerves in both the brain and body be more responsive to our complex world. BDNF tends to be low in people with anxiety.

In summary, when you miss meals or skip the protein in meals, and rely on just carbohydrates to fuel your body and brain, a number of uncomfortable things can happen. Symptoms of anxiety increase because of the adrenaline released into your body and brain. Without enough fuel from meals and snacks, you use muscle mass as a glucose source, effectively decreasing your muscle mass, which supports both physical and mental health.

At this point, you might be thinking that you want to eat regular meals and get regular exercise—but you may be worrying about how you'll fit all that into your schedule or how you can stick with the changes you'd like to make even when things get stressful. We assure you that what we're going to ask you to try is doable, without causing real disruptions to your routines. And it will help reduce your anxiety and fatigue.

PHYSIOLOGY OF ANXIETY IN A NUTSHELL

In the first two chapters, the "Snapshot of Anxiety Assessment" and "What Impacts Anxiety" worksheet helped you determine your particular pattern of symptoms. This chapter focuses on physiology and explains how food choices can actually create the symptoms of worry, anxiety, and fatigue. We explained how one and a half to two hours after a low-fiber, high-carbohydrate food, like cereal or a bagel, blood glucose levels drop, and the brain starts to worry about its fuel supply and releases adrenaline to signal that the body urgently needs to make its own glucose. To correct the low glucose supply quickly, we have to eat carbohydrates or our body will make glucose from its own protein source—muscle.

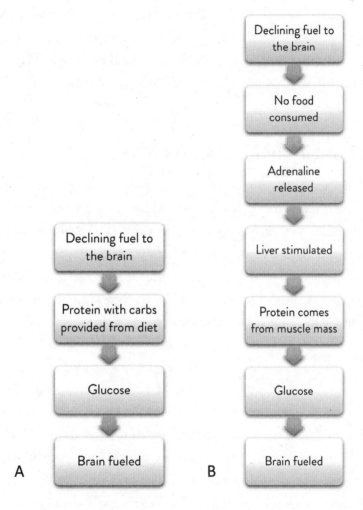

A. Fuel for the body and brain are provided through a balanced meal or snack that contains protein and carbs. Glucose from the food fuels the brain.

B. Going long hours without food, the brain demands fuel from the body, adrenaline is released, stimulating the liver to make glucose from protein, which ultimately comes from muscle mass to fuel the body. For more on the physiology, see a video explaining the physiology at http://www.newharbinger.com/46233.

The ideal scenario would be to eat some carbohydrates *with* protein. If we don't eat some quick fuel, the rush of adrenaline shifts our brains into survival mode before the protein (a slower, more stable fuel) can be utilized. The release of adrenaline immediately and adversely impacts our cognition, our emotions, and our choices. Specifically, adrenaline shifts us from the responsive-cortex brain into the reactive-limbic system. The limbic system responds to the things you encounter with fight behaviors (like irritation), flight behaviors (like anxiety), disappear behaviors (such as checking out, bingeing on sugar or social media, or isolating), or default behaviors (past emotional reactions and behaviors). Additionally, the effect of adrenaline on the body mimics anxiety by causing a racing heart, increased respiration, and tense muscles, among other symptoms. Because this ancient lizard brain is focused only on survival, we're no longer able to respond to the world in a thoughtful way.

Phew! You've made it through the hardest science. Let's put all this back into Luca's life and see if it's familiar.

Luca Forgets to Go to the Grocery Store

During breakfast, Luca notices there's nothing in the refrigerator to eat for dinner and makes a mental note to go to the grocery store after work. At midday, her responsive-cortex brain remembers that she needs to go to the grocery store after work. Luca then eats lunch: spaghetti with red sauce and a small salad. By 3:00 p.m., her brain is beginning to run out of fuel, and her body decides to make its own fuel to feed her brain by releasing adrenaline and other hormones that help the liver produce the needed glucose. By 5:00 p.m., there's enough adrenaline in her system that the reactive-limbic brain is fully in charge. She notes that some of her work emails are making her distressed. Rather than answering them, she avoids them—thinking she will reply to them from home, before she goes to bed. Instead of going to the grocery store, Luca drives home because that route is familiar, comfortable, and habitual. Her low-glucose, adrenaline-flooded reactive-limbic brain uses the default behavior, which is to go home.

When Kristen is in that situation, she can get herself to drive to the grocery store by repeating, "Go to the grocery store, go to the grocery store." Once she makes the turn away from home to the store, she's okay; she's now in a different default behavior—driving to the grocery store. However, it took a lot of effort to focus her mind and call upon her responsive-cortex brain to override her reactive-limbic brain to turn away from home and go to the grocery store.

Of course, when she gets there, she's going to be focused on foods laden with salt, sugar, and fat since the reactive-limbic system is genetically programmed to focus on these foods. Kristen might even "forget" to purchase healthy foods. Adrenaline has her in survival mode. Loud and persuasive, the reactive-limbic brain convinces her to buy the sugary, fatty food. "Ice cream will help me, right? YES!!" screams the inner committee, "ICE CREAM!!"

Alternatively, when she's fed and at the grocery store, she's in her smart responsive-cortex brain, and it's easier to tune out the request for treats. She can focus on buying foods that she enjoys and that are supportive for her body and brain.

Because Luca had mostly carbohydrates with very little protein for lunch, she's teetering on the edge of pre-explosive physiology. Just as she pulls into her driveway, she remembers that she meant to go to the grocery store on her way home. Sitting in the car, trying to decide if she is going to go inside or to the store, Luca's phone rings. She sees that it's her boss and picks up. Her boss is calling because one of their clients is hoping to get a face-to-face update on their project tomorrow at 10:00 a.m. Luca's boss wants to know if she can make the meeting. Her boss assures her that she just needs to give a short update and answer questions, and makes it clear that she doesn't expect Luca to prepare a formal presentation on such short notice. At this moment, Luca's responsive-cortex brain is grateful for the opportunity to meet the client in person and hears that her boss is being supportive. Luca says yes.

But the minute she gets off the phone, she loses it. Luca's body starts to tremble, and she can't catch her breath; her hands are shaking as she unhooks the seatbelt. At first, she just stares ahead. Her panic is rising. Her body is producing even more adrenaline than before the phone call. Where a few moments before she could access the responsive-cortex part of her brain to engage with her boss, that's now becoming increasingly impossible. Luca's mind is racing with thoughts that are not organized at all. The one clear voice in her head is the voice of her mother telling her that she's too stupid to meet with the client or give the presentation. The voice starts to catastrophize, telling her that she'll do horribly and be responsible for losing her client. Additionally, maybe her boss is setting her up for failure. In this moment, with the adrenaline and depleting glucose levels preventing her from thinking with her responsive-cortex brain (and causing her to default to her reactive-limbic brain), Luca can't hold on to the fact that her boss is setting her up for success and a possible promotion. Her boss is giving her an opportunity to do what will be expected in the new position. But her reactive-limbic brain is just playing all the default records stored for survival, which don't support her in being at her best. What she chooses next in terms of fueling her brain will impact what happens for the rest of the evening, how she sleeps, and if she'll be at her best the next morning.

We are going to hit the pause button on this story for a couple of reasons. First, we don't need to go into any more detail about Luca's resulting panic attack—those adrenaline-induced feelings are almost jumping off the page! Also, we're wondering if you recognize this moment. Has anything like this happened to you? Can you see how not being fueled is escalating this moment for Luca?

Is there a situation in your life that triggers symptoms of anxiety that you would like to change? Take a few minutes to jot down some things that you would like to do if your anxiety didn't get in the way.

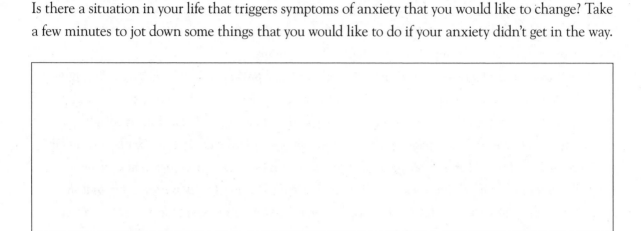

The next section explains how you can use the physiology we've been exploring to reduce the worry, anxiety, and fatigue that keep you from achieving the objectives you've written about. When it comes to addressing your anxiety and getting back on track toward your life goals, knowing the why improves your ability to engage with the what and how.

THE PROTEIN SOLUTION (PROTEIN WITH CARBS)

In this section, you'll learn how small frequent meals and snacks with protein and carbohydrates reduce the adrenaline that triggers your symptoms. This approach keeps your glucose levels stable throughout the day. You might have heard this solution before. Maybe you tried it for a reason other than reducing anxiety and fatigue. Perhaps you noticed that you felt better, but your other goal didn't materialize the way that you were hoping it would, so you stopped. This time, the focus is on being at your best. Using food to feel better in a sustainable way can be a total lifestyle changer. Or, it can be something you sometimes do because you really, *really*, REALLY need to not meltdown with anxiety.

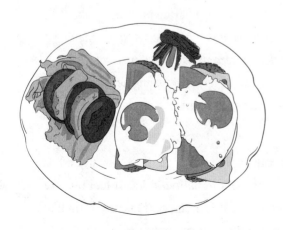

When you eat *protein with carbohydrates* instead of just carbohydrates, your brain has fuel for three to four hours instead of one and a half to two hours. By doing this small thing, you double the time that your responsive-cortex brain is in charge! Under this condition, any adrenaline in your system is probably caused by external reasons, and you'll likely know what's causing you distress. You can say, "That is making me anxious." When anxiety occurs for physiological reasons, you might feel more like, "I'm anxious, and I don't know why."

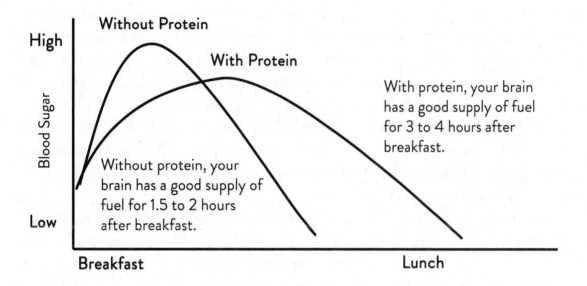

Comparing Breakfasts With and Without Protein

Let's put it this way: Imagine that you had to spend your days in a room with no windows and the lights were controlled by a timer. You have two options for the lights to be on: (1) use a switch in the room to keep the lights on for one and a half to two hours or (2) walk out of the room and down the hall to another switch that keeps the lights on for three to four hours. The switch that is further away takes a little more effort, but the benefit lasts longer. In reality, some days you would likely use the switch in the room, and other days you'd opt for the extended benefit. It would probably depend on what was happening day-to-day. Would you take the time to walk down the hall if you wanted to do something with less disruption and you needed more than two hours to get it done?

Because adrenaline isn't released as quickly after a protein-rich meal with carbohydrates, you get more time in the responsive-cortex part of your brain, with the reactive-limbic system firmly in the backseat. By having protein with meals and snacks, you'll feel less anxiety and more energy throughout the day.

We'll discuss how much protein to eat in the next chapter. For now, all you need to know is that when you eat protein with some carbohydrates, your brain has fuel for a longer time. This is an important point: you need *protein with some carbohydrates*. Let's think about why this is. If your brain is running out of glucose and you only eat protein, say jerky or turkey, will your brain have immediate access to glucose? No. Will you get an adrenaline release even though you just ate? Yes. Remember, this is because carbohydrates supply the quick fuel and protein supplies the stable, longer-lasting fuel.

Sydney started working with Kristen because she wanted to reduce her anxiety. Sydney was panicking and crying midmorning and midafternoon every day in the bathroom at work. When Kristen asked her what she ate most days, she said that she had protein bars for breakfast and lunch, and some kind of meat with rice and butter and a salad for dinner. Kristen asked her if there were times when she was not anxious, and after thinking about it, Sydney said in the evenings. Kristen asked if she liked her work. Sydney explained she did for a long time, but over the last few months, she didn't because her anxiety was getting worse at work. She couldn't think of a good reason for the change. Kristen asked what kind of protein bar she was eating, and Sydney showed her the bar. It had lots of protein but no real carbohydrate, and though it was branded as a bar that was low in sugar, all the sweetness it did have came from artificial sugars.

Sydney thought she was doing a good thing by choosing a bar with less sugar, but it wasn't giving her brain what it needed—an appropriate amount of glucose—so she was anxious and tired at work. What's more, even a protein bar with artificial sugars will still trigger an insulin release—many people's bodies release insulin when the nose and taste buds detect sweetness—which would usher the small amount of blood glucose that *was* in her bloodstream into the cells. This crash in her glucose levels was the cause of her symptoms. Meanwhile, she felt better in the evenings because her meal had the four basics: protein (meat), carbohydrate (rice), fat (butter and oil in the salad dressing), and fiber (salad).

To address her problems, Kristen replaced Sydney's protein bars with a bar that had a ratio of two parts carbohydrates to one part protein (about 24 grams of carbs to 12 grams of protein), and she immediately felt better. Kristen hoped that as Sydney recovered, she would plan meals with real foods for breakfast and lunch, as small consistent steps can lead to bigger changes over time. Now that Sydney understood the physiology and had the tools to make better decisions, Kristen knew she would find her own path.

BACK TO LUCA

When we left Luca's story, Luca was in her driveway. She hadn't had much protein for breakfast or lunch and had forgotten to go to the grocery store on her way home. This set up the physiological conditions for her panic attack after her boss called and asked her to meet with a client the next morning.

What if we could roll back time, and Luca had had three meatballs with her spaghetti lunch? First, there is a greater chance that Luca would have been at the grocery store when her boss called. She would have been more in the responsive-cortex part of her brain and been able to hold on to the fact that her boss was giving her an opportunity. She may have still gotten anxious, but there's less likelihood that she would have had a full-blown panic attack. Plus, when she was at the store, she might have gotten her favorite sweet treat. If Luca is like many others, she would have eaten her treat in the car while thinking—maybe even worrying a little bit—about what she needs to do before her 10:00 a.m. meeting with her client. But with this influx of quick fuel, after twenty minutes, Luca's brain would have given the signal that everything was okay. And if Luca had dinner within an hour or so, she would avoid getting another adrenaline hit when she burned through the fuel from her treat.

Let's also pause to wash away some guilt. Luca might feel as if she had no self-control because, under stress, she "caved" and ate her favorite treat. Yes, eating lots of treats can cause anxiety, depression, and physical health consequences. However, it's also a way to manage anxiety and keep the responsive-cortex part of the brain in charge of thoughts and emotions until a full meal can be had. If you struggle with cravings when you're stressed, this is your brain asking for fuel, and feeding your brain is a form of self-care! While it does have consequences if done repeatedly over time, in the short term, it can help while you learn new tools that will reduce your reliance on treats.

REFLECTIONS

Can you think of some examples of when your physiology contributes to your symptoms of anxiety, worry, and fatigue? What are some things that you might do differently? Use the space below to write or draw it out in your own words.

CHAPTER SUMMARY

Now that you have some understanding of how your physiology impacts how you interact with who and what is happening around you, we're going to give you detailed solutions for reducing anxiety, worry, and fatigue. If watching videos or listening to podcasts explaining the physiology would be helpful, you can find them at http://www.kristenallott.com. When you understand the importance of fueling your brain, you can start to shift the symptoms you listed in the Snapshot of Anxiety Assessment and improve the patterns you identified in the What Impacts Anxiety worksheet.

Next, in chapters 4 to 7, we'll cover:

- How to set yourself up for success the next day

- How to get through high-stakes events (like Luca's presentation) at your best

- What to do if you wake up with racing thoughts, worries, or memories of nightmares

- How to have sustained energy throughout the day.

Part II

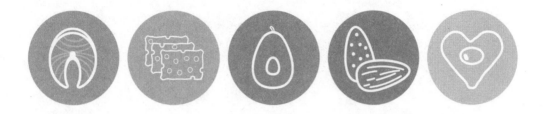

Protein Experiments
for You to Try

## CHAPTER 4

A Three-Day Protein Experiment

In the fast pace of today's world, we all want to have more energy and mental clarity. Many of us get paid for our ability to think and make effective decisions within a tight timeline or schedule. Studies show that our ability to concentrate, have self-control, assess a situation, and creatively problem solve for good decision making is determined in large part by the physical resources of our brains—our power supply. Small frequent meals that contain protein and carbohydrates help stabilize blood glucose to help you feel better. Over the long term, it's also important to eat vegetables, fruits, healthy fat, and whole grains to keep your whole body healthy.

In this chapter, we'll experiment with increasing your protein intake throughout the day, in both meals and snacks. It's helpful to start the process of changing your dietary fuel with adjustments to your protein intake, in particular, because it's easier to *add* what's missing than to *restrict* habitual foods. We're here to make you feel better, not worse, and to make your life easier, not harder! With that, let's get started.

THE THREE-DAY PROTEIN EXPERIMENT TO STABILIZE GLUCOSE AND REDUCE ANXIETY

For three days, try adding protein to your meals and snacks over the course of each day. Here is a template to give you ideas, which you can adjust to meet your dietary preferences and needs; we'll give you more examples of how you might tailor your meals and snacks to make them interesting.

Example Diet

7:00 a.m.	**Breakfast** (14 g protein): ideally within an hour of waking, two eggs, one piece of toast, one apple or pear.
10:00 a.m.	**Snack** (6–7 g protein): ¼ cup of nuts (choose from almonds, peanuts, cashews, hazelnuts) or ¼ cup of cottage cheese or 2 tbsp of nut butter (peanut, almond, or cashew).
12:00–1:00 p.m.	**Lunch** (21 g protein): portion of meat the size of a deck of cards. This can be eaten as a sandwich, wrap, salad, or soup. Plus 1 cup of veggies and/or 1 cup of whole grains (such as brown rice, quinoa, bulgur). Be sure that you consume a little bit of veggie fat as well, such as avocado, nut oil, or olive oil.
3:00 p.m.	**Snack** (6–7 g protein): ¼ cup of nuts: (choose from almonds, peanuts, cashews, hazelnuts), or ¼ cup of cottage cheese, or 2 tbsp of nut butter (peanut, almond, or cashew).
6:00 p.m.	**Dinner** (21 g protein): portion of meat the size of a deck of cards. This can be eaten as a sandwich, wrap, salad, or soup. Plus 1 cup of veggies or 1 cup of whole grains (such as brown rice, quinoa, bulgur). Be sure that you consume a little bit of veggie fat as well, such as avocado, nut oil, or olive oil.
Before bed:	(6–7 g protein): 1–2 slices of turkey meat. *Note: This is a suggestion for people who have difficulty staying asleep throughout the night or who have nightmares; we explain how this works in chapter 7: "Fueling Your Brain for Better Sleep."*

Most people can feel a difference in their energy and mental clarity within three days of eating enough protein. The three-day experiment is based on a target protein intake of 68–76 grams daily.

Based on USDA recommended daily allowances, the quick calculation for your target protein intake is 8 grams of protein for every 20 pounds of body weight (with a maximum of 120 grams of protein per day). Use the chart to find your ideal range of daily protein.

Your Weight (lb)	Target (g protein)	Acceptable Range (g protein)
100	40	36–45
120	48	43–54
140	56	50–63
160	64	57–72
180	72	64–81
200	80	71–90

Kristen has observed that most people, regardless of weight, do better if they are getting at least 65 grams of protein over the course of a day. Unless your weight is below 120 pounds, we suggest that 65–80 grams of protein per day is a good place to start. For those under 120 pounds, scale the protein in the example diet to 40–48 grams. If you're over 200 pounds, 65 grams of protein throughout the day is still enough to start reducing the physiological causes of your anxiety and fatigue. If you want to experiment with eating more protein, we recommend capping the amount of protein at 120 grams unless you're working closely with a health care provider. If you're gluten-free or have other dietary restrictions, modify the example diet as appropriate. *This amount of protein is safe for most people, unless you have kidney disease or a metabolic condition that restricts your ability to process protein. Please consult with your doctor before changing your diet.*

To help you customize your experiment, we've created a chart that shows the amount of protein in different foods. The amounts of protein provided may vary depending on type or brand. If in doubt, refer to the label of the food you're eating. Remember to note the grams of protein per serving size so that you're still meeting your target.

Healthy Protein Sources

Meat

Meat (poultry, beef, pork, lamb): 3 oz = 21 g

Farmed or wild fish: 3 oz = 21 g

Eggs

Egg, whole: 1 egg = 7 g

Egg substitute: ¼ c = 7 g

Egg white: 1 = 4 g

Note: You might be tempted to go with egg whites whenever possible to avoid having yolks. But egg yolks contain nutrients that are excellent for mental health.

Legumes

Tofu: ½ c = 10 g

Tempeh: ½ c = 16 g

Lentils: ½ c = 9 g

Refried beans: ½ c = 8 g

Whole beans: ½ c = 7 g

Nuts & Seeds

Nuts: ¼ c = 8 g

Nut butter: 2 tbsp = 8 g

Seed butter: 2 tbsp = 5 g

Seeds: 2 tbsp = 3 g

Seed Grains

Quinoa: ½ c = 11 g

Barley: ½ c = 10 g

Dark rye flour: ½ c = 9 g

Millet: ½ c = 4 g

Oats: ½ c = 3 g

Brown rice: ½ c = 3 g

White rice: ½ c = 3 g

Dairy Substitutes

Soy milk: 1 c = 6 g

Soy cheese: 1 oz = 4–7 g

Soy yogurt: 1 c = 6 g

Note: Nut milks often don't contain substantial amounts of protein.

Dairy

Cottage cheese: ½ c = 12 g

Yogurt: 1 c = 8–14 g

Other

Protein powder: 1 tbsp = 9–20 g

Plant-based meat substitutes: 9–17 g

You may have noticed that milk and cheese are not on this list. While these are sources of protein for children, in her clinical practice, Kristen has found through bloodwork that they don't have the same physiological impact in most adults. These may still be a part of your overall diet, but we don't recommend that you count them toward your daily protein target. If you really like milk or cheese *as a protein source*, do an experiment: eat a cheese sandwich (or the like) for three days to see if it maintains your energy level as effectively as other protein sources. If the protein source works for you, great! But you may find that in order to get the extra support you need, it can be really helpful to understand the place that particular foods have in your diet.

It also helps, when you're adding protein—or anything new—to your diet, to think about portion control. Here are some visual clues to help you keep your servings to the proper size:

- 3 oz of meat = a deck of playing cards

- 1 c yogurt = a hand holding a tennis ball

- ½ c cooked grain and beans = a small fist

- 1 oz cheese = a thumb

- 1 oz nuts = a golf ball

- 1 tbsp nut butter or nuts = a silver dollar or a walnut

- 1 tsp oil = a quarter

SETTING UP AN EXPERIMENT

When setting up an experiment, we recommend that you:

- Have an idea of what you want to get from it,

- Understand the steps to get there,

- Understand how long you need to do the experiment to reasonably expect results (*Hint: experiments in this workbook take anywhere from 30 seconds to 30 days to deliver results*), and then

- Ask yourself if you got the results you hoped for.

The most important criterion for determining the success of an experiment is to ask, *Do I feel better?* at the end of it. Changing your behavior patterns can be uncomfortable, even scary; we all have a certain amount of drive to keep things as they are, even if we're not particularly happy about it. And we all understand that if we don't feel like something's actually working for us, we're not likely to keep it up. Keeping track of it and how much better you feel will help you compensate for these realities and decide if it's worth putting in the energy to sustain the new behavior.

EXPERIMENT: TRY THREE DAYS OF MEALS AND SNACKS WITH PROTEIN

Set aside three continuous days to try this experiment. For three days, keep track of your protein intake, how you feel, and how much energy you have. (Note that some people may not observe a difference until they go back to their normal diet and notice that they feel worse.)

Start date (day 1): _____

Step 1: At the *beginning* of the first day, circle the numbers that best indicate the range of your power supply and anxiety level over the last week.

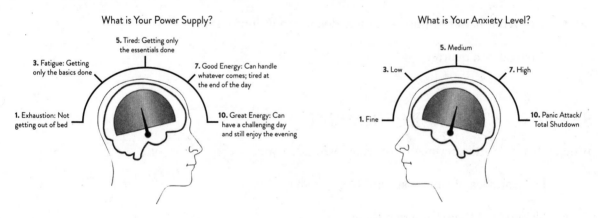

Step 2: Follow or adapt the example diet provided earlier in this chapter. Write down the sources and approximate quantities of protein you eat throughout the day.

Time: _____ Breakfast: _____

_____

Amount of protein eaten: _____

Time: _____ Snack: _____

_____

Amount of protein eaten: _____

Time: _____ Lunch: _____

_____

Amount of protein eaten: _____

Time: _____ Snack: _____

_____

Amount of protein eaten: _____

Time: _____ Dinner: _____

_____

Amount of protein eaten: _____

Time: _____ Before Bed: _____

_____

Amount of protein eaten: _____

Step 3: At the *end* of the first day, circle the numbers that best indicate your power supply and anxiety level. Make notes about any other changes to how you feel.

What is Your Power Supply?

5. Tired: Getting only the essentials done

3. Fatigue: Getting only the basics done

7. Good Energy: Can handle whatever comes; tired at the end of the day

1. Exhaustion: Not getting out of bed

10. Great Energy: Can have a challenging day and still enjoy the evening

What is Your Anxiety Level?

5. Medium

3. Low

7. High

1. Fine

10. Panic Attack/ Total Shutdown

Day 2: _____

Step 1: At the *beginning* of the second day, circle the numbers that best indicate the range of your power supply and anxiety level over the last week.

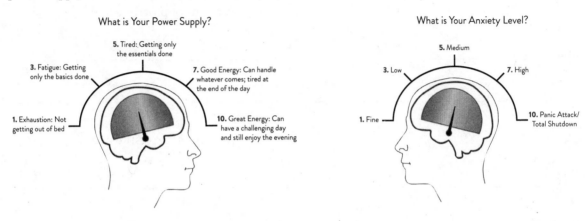

What is Your Power Supply?

3. Fatigue: Getting only the basics done

5. Tired: Getting only the essentials done

7. Good Energy: Can handle whatever comes; tired at the end of the day

1. Exhaustion: Not getting out of bed

10. Great Energy: Can have a challenging day and still enjoy the evening

What is Your Anxiety Level?

3. Low

5. Medium

7. High

1. Fine

10. Panic Attack/ Total Shutdown

Step 2: Follow or adapt the example diet provided earlier in this chapter. Write down the sources and approximate quantities of protein you eat throughout the day.

Time: _____ Breakfast: _____

_____

Amount of protein eaten: _____

Time: _____ Snack: _____

_____

Amount of protein eaten: _____

Time: _____ Lunch: _____

_____

Amount of protein eaten: _____

Time: _____ Snack: _____

_____

Amount of protein eaten: _____

Time: _____ Dinner: _____

_____

Amount of protein eaten: _____

Time: _____ Before Bed: _____

_____

Amount of protein eaten: _____

Step 3: At the *end* of the second day, circle the numbers that best indicate your power supply and anxiety level. Make notes about any other changes to how you feel.

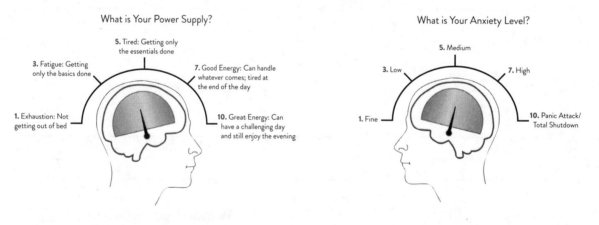

[ ]

Day 3: _____

Step 1: At the *beginning* of the third day, circle the numbers that best indicate the range of your power supply and anxiety level over the last week.

What is Your Power Supply?

5. Tired: Getting only the essentials done

3. Fatigue: Getting only the basics done

7. Good Energy: Can handle whatever comes; tired at the end of the day

1. Exhaustion: Not getting out of bed

10. Great Energy: Can have a challenging day and still enjoy the evening

What is Your Anxiety Level?

5. Medium

3. Low

7. High

1. Fine

10. Panic Attack/ Total Shutdown

Step 2: Follow or adapt the example diet provided earlier in this chapter. Write down the sources and approximate quantities of protein you eat throughout the day.

Time: _____ Breakfast: _____

_____

Amount of protein eaten: _____

Time: _____ Snack: _____

_____

Amount of protein eaten: _____

Time: _____ Lunch: _____

_____

Amount of protein eaten: _____

Time: _____ Snack: _____

_____

Amount of protein eaten: _____

Time: _____ Dinner: _____

_____

Amount of protein eaten: _____

Time: _____ Before Bed: _____

_____

Amount of protein eaten: _____

Step 3: At the *end* of the third day, circle the numbers that best indicate your power supply and anxiety level. Make notes about any other changes to how you feel.

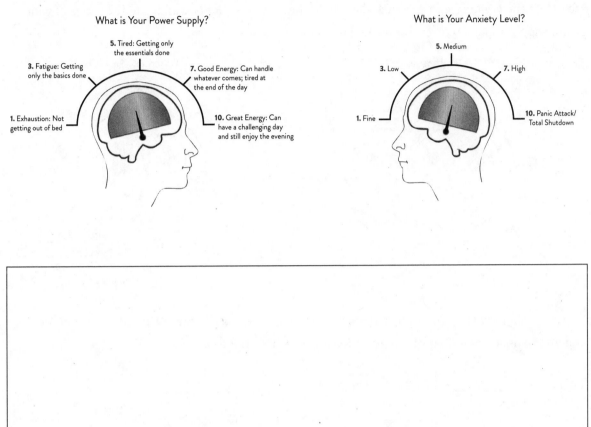

What is Your Power Supply?

5. Tired: Getting only the essentials done

3. Fatigue: Getting only the basics done

7. Good Energy: Can handle whatever comes; tired at the end of the day

1. Exhaustion: Not getting out of bed

10. Great Energy: Can have a challenging day and still enjoy the evening

What is Your Anxiety Level?

5. Medium

3. Low

7. High

1. Fine

10. Panic Attack/ Total Shutdown

Day 4 (optional): _____

Step 1: At the *beginning* of the fourth day, circle the numbers that best indicate the range of your power supply and anxiety level over the last week.

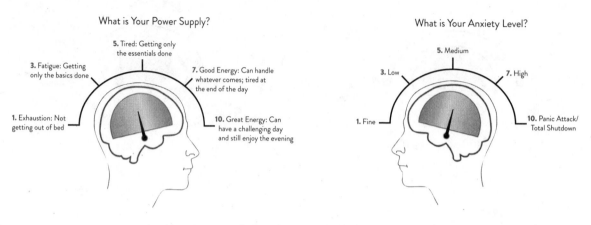

Step 2: Follow or adapt the example diet provided earlier in this chapter. Write down the sources and approximate quantities of protein you eat throughout the day.

Time: _____ Breakfast: _____

_____

Amount of protein eaten: _____

Time: _____ Snack: _____

_____

Amount of protein eaten: _____

Time: _____ Lunch: _____

_____

Amount of protein eaten: _____

Time: _____ Snack: _____

_____

Amount of protein eaten: _____

Time: _____ Dinner: _____

_____

Amount of protein eaten: _____

Time: _____ Before Bed: _____

_____

Amount of protein eaten: _____

Step 3: At the *end* of the fourth day, circle the numbers that best indicate your power supply and anxiety level. Make notes about any other changes to how you feel.

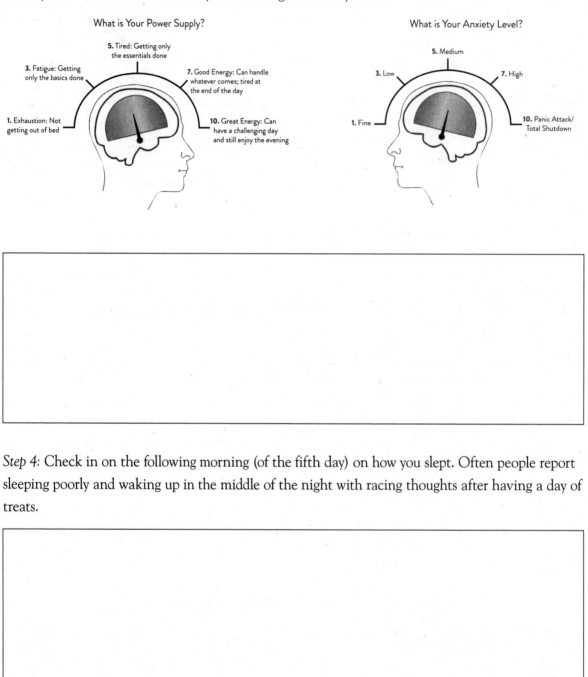

Step 4: Check in on the following morning (of the fifth day) on how you slept. Often people report sleeping poorly and waking up in the middle of the night with racing thoughts after having a day of treats.

REFLECTIONS

Write down your reflections about whether it was hard to reach your daily protein target. What made it challenging or easy? Did known anxiety triggers come up during the three days? How did you respond?

Remember that tending to your fuel supply will ease some, but not necessarily all, of your symptoms of anxiety. If you still experienced anxiety, you might have noticed a change in the quality or symptoms. Depending on your relationship with your body, you might not be able to notice a difference until you go back to your old diet and recognize that you don't feel so good or have more difficulty managing your anxiety, worry, and fatigue. Whatever your experience, it's okay! This workbook is geared toward helping you better understand yourself.

CHAPTER SUMMARY

Doing experiments is the best way to notice what effects behavioral factors, like diet, might have on the level of anxiety you feel. The Three-Day Protein Experiment Tracking Worksheet is available for download at http://www.newharbinger.com/46233.

In the next, chapter we'll explore reading labels to help you find the foods that will give you more energy and mental clarity.

## CHAPTER 5

Understanding Food Labels: Eating for Increased Energy and Mental Clarity

Do you know what you're eating? Do you believe that the food industry knows about your personal health? This chapter teaches you how to evaluate nutritional labels on the foods you consume and which components are the most important for supporting energy and mental clarity.

When Kristen was in school at Bastyr University, she wanted to understand labels on packaged food. She thought that when she read a label, she should be able to understand what kind of fuel was going into her body and how it would make her *feel*. But first Kristen had to know which information on the label she needed to pay attention to. She was confused at first about the difference between total carbohydrates and sugars. Kristen thought that they should be the same, or at least add up, but they usually don't. What she found is that a whole bunch of history, committee meetings, lobbying, bureaucracy, and other nonnutritional sagas goes into a food label. Someone…not us…could write a book about all that. In the sections that follow, you'll learn to close-read nutrition facts and food labels to figure out what you're eating and what effect it will have on your anxiety and your energy levels.

COMPONENTS OF A FOOD LABEL

Hopefully, we're all at least a little familiar with the nutrition facts labels on the back of all packaged food in the US. The label usually starts with *serving size*. The nutrition facts provided represent what is in the reported serving size. It's important to adjust the nutrition facts to correspond to the amount that you actually eat. This is an important factor to keep in mind when trying to understand what you're actually getting from a meal or snack.

Based on the listed serving size, the label then reports on:

- Calories (and calories from fat)

- The amounts of fat, cholesterol, sodium, total carbohydrates, and protein, as well as particular vitamins and minerals

- The calculations of percentage of daily value, based on a 2,000-calorie diet. This provides a general idea of how much of the different nutritional components are in the food in relation to the recommended daily allowance, per USDA guidance.

And then the ingredients are typically listed, either below or next to the nutrition facts.

HOW TO READ A LABEL FOR REDUCED ANXIETY, INCREASED ENERGY, AND MENTAL CLARITY

There can be different goals for choosing the foods we eat, and these goals impact how we interpret food labels. For example:

- Are we trying to make "healthier choices"? This goal often changes with the latest news or fads.

- Are we concerned about lower cholesterol levels? In this case, we are often taught to look at fiber or fat content, and perhaps total carbs or sugars.

- Are we trying to lose weight? Historically, calories are what we think of, sometimes ignoring the rest of the label.

- Are we concerned about high blood pressure? Salt, or sodium content, is often what we look for.

The food industry understands that most people think in these broader categories and are savvy in their marketing on the front of the package—"Low Cal," "Low Fat," "Low Sodium," "High Fiber," or whatever the current trend may be. Many of us look for these key words on the front of the packaging and skip the food label altogether. The type of food we eat plays a huge role in how we *feel* and when we'll want to eat again. It also significantly impacts our energy levels, mental clarity, and our ability to cope with stressful situations. While these other things aren't unimportant, the key words on food packaging don't tell us much about the impact the foods will have on our energy and mental clarity within two to four hours after eating.

Let's look at a label to assess what our energy level will be in two to four hours after eating the food, or until the next meal or snack. Let's use a common breakfast cereal, as an example.

Step 1: Determine how much protein is in a serving. This particular cereal has 3 grams of protein per serving.

Step 2: Note the calories per serving. Many diet programs focus exclusively on calorie intake even though science has shown that the "calories in, calories out" formula does not lead to weight loss or improved health. Still, we are so trained to look at calories per serving that I don't want to take away this step. For this cereal, there are 95 calories in ¾ cup.

Step 3: Look at the serving size and servings per container. The serving size directly relates to all the other components. Here, it's ¾ cup of cereal. Three-quarters of a cup of cereal doesn't seem very realistic, but this is an area where the food industry likes to play games.

In essence, the important part of reading a label is to use the information provided to calculate what you're *really* taking in. In this example, there are 3 grams of protein in ¾ cup, so if you have three servings (2¼ cups), you're actually getting 9 grams of protein. The same is true, of course, for calories. If there are 95 calories per serving and you eat three servings, you're actually consuming 285 calories.

Step 4: Calculate the carbohydrates. A carbohydrate is a molecule that is made up of sugars, starch, and cellulose. When we have a meal, most people need to have some digestible carbohydrates—our bodies absorb the sugars from the carbohydrates

Nutrition Facts	
About 24 servings per container	
Serving size	**¾ cup (30g)**
Amount per serving	
Calories	**95**
	% Daily Value*
Total Fat 0.5g	1%
Saturated Fat 0g	
Trans Fat	
Polyunsaturated Fat	
Monounsaturated Fat	
Cholesterol 0mg	0%
Sodium 240mg	6%
Total Carbohydrate 24g	8%
Dietary Fiber 4g	15%
Soluble Fiber 1g	
Insoluble Fiber 3g	
Total Sugars 10g	
Includes 4g Added Sugars	9%
Protein 3g	

*The % Daily Value (DV) tells you how much a nutrient in a serving of food contributes to a daily diet. 2,000 calories a day is used for general nutrition advice.

and use them as fuel (glucose). In fact, the nerves of our brain *need* glucose; remember that glucose tells our brain that everything is okay. This is why we're attracted to eating foods with carbohydrates. The problem is that often the foods we eat are too high in carbohydrates. This spikes our glucose—and helps us be more emotionally comfortable in the short term—but high-carb foods don't have the fuel to keep us in our responsive-cortex brains for long, so we inevitably crash. When we start to crash—generally about two hours after a high-carb meal—we typically don't associate it with the bagel we ate at 8:00 a.m.

But avoiding all carbohydrates isn't the answer either; this can cause fatigue, anxiety, and irritability. Rather, the aim is to get the right *ratio* of carbohydrates to protein—a ratio that will provide more energy and mental clarity, keep us from being as reactive to our emotions and our anxiety, and leave us physically healthier and more emotionally stable. Fueling your body so you stay in your responsive-cortex brain is a more effective way of achieving those goals than eliminating carbs altogether.

For our purposes here, there are two parts to understanding how the amount of carbohydrates in food will affect your mood. The first is to understand what *calculated carbs* are and how to get this number. The "total carbohydrates" figure you'll see on the standard nutrition facts label is based on the number of calories released by burning the food in a laboratory setting. There are often two subcomponents listed in total carbohydrates on a label: dietary fiber (and sometimes insoluble fiber) and sugars. And you'll notice that these never add up to the total carb number.

Calculated carbs, on the other hand, are the total carbs minus the fiber(s) that tends to skew the total carbohydrate figure. Dietary and insoluble fiber are used by the bacteria in your gut to keep your gut healthy. They move right through your gut, become stool, and are expelled. For the most part, fiber is not used as calories to fuel your body, which is why we don't include them in the calculated carbs.

The lines in the label under "Total Carbohydrate" that say "Total Sugars" or "Other Carbohydrates" are a bit more ambiguous. For sugars, the label doesn't tell us what kind of sugars and is based on a bureaucratic calculation rather than nutritional information. For the purpose of determining how you're likely to feel after eating the food product, you can simply ignore (but not subtract) these lines.

So, in our cereal example, there are 20 calculated carbs—24 grams (total carbs) minus 4 grams (total dietary fiber).

When we're thinking about how we'll feel after eating a food, it's this calculated carb number—considered with the amount of protein—that we're interested in. And that brings us to the second part of understanding why calculated carbs are so important, step 5.

Step 5: Find the calculated-carb-to-protein ratio. The real effect of carbohydrates on mood is understood through the calculated-carb-to-protein ratio. In our cereal example, there are 20 grams of calculated carbs to 3 grams of protein, which is a ratio of roughly 7:1. Note that this ratio doesn't change with the number of servings you consume.

Calculated-carb-to-protein ratios of 1:1 to 4:1 will have the effect of eating a healthy balance of protein and carbohydrates. Glucose levels will be stable, and you'll have energy, even if it's a snack and not a full meal. Ratios around 5:1 to 7:1 fall in the "dessert" range: you'll get a quicker hit of glucose but will crash more quickly as well. We consider ratios greater than 7:1 as a "sugar rush": stuff that's fun to have in the moment but will most likely make you feel crappy later.

With all this in mind, this cereal alone won't likely sustain you through the morning!

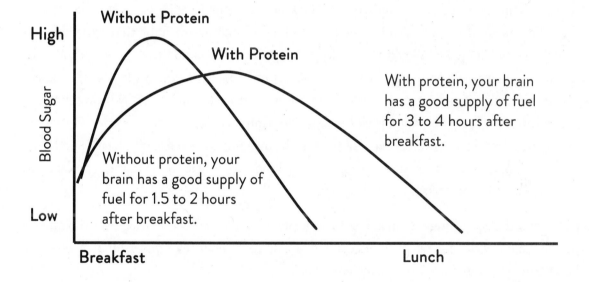

Comparing Breakfasts With and Without Protein

Let's think about why this is true: About two hours after eating cereal or any other simple, low-fiber, high-carbohydrate food for breakfast or any other meal or snack, blood glucose levels drop, and the brain starts to worry about its fuel supplies. This, in turn, triggers the release of hormones to make glucose, including adrenaline. The release of adrenaline immediately impacts how we make decisions, we're more reactive emotionally, our bodies have more fatigue, and we crave sugar. When this happens repeatedly, muscle mass is broken down into amino acids. Those amino acids are then converted into glucose by the liver, some of which becomes stored in our fat cells. As muscle mass diminishes, our metabolic rates decline, and we become less able to eat the same number of calories without increasing our weight and size. We also increase the likelihood of developing type 2 diabetes. Unfortunately, there are even more undesirable effects than those aforementioned.

The calculated-carb-to-protein ratio is the key to understanding how foods will affect our mental clarity, energy, and mood, and we'll return to this later in this chapter. But first let's touch on the fats section of the nutrition label and the ingredient list to round out our understanding of how to really assess the quality of the foods we're eating.

Step 6: Identify the types of fats. We need healthy fat in our diet because fat makes up the cellular membrane of every cell in our bodies, including our brains. Fats are the backbone of steroid hormones (the messenger system of the body), and they're also the source of fuel our muscles prefer to burn when we engage in sufficient movement. But not all fats are the same. In addition to noting the amount of fat in the product, it's important to look at the ingredient list (step 7) to understand whether the fats are from animals or vegetables. Animal fats are less healthy than vegetable fats. Saturated fats and trans fats should be avoided, since saturated fats and trans fats in shelf-stable foods, such as margarine, contribute to cardiovascular disease and dementia. So, look at the ingredient list of the foods you buy so you can avoid shortenings, trans fats, and partially hydrogenated or hydrogenated oils. And what if the package says "No Trans Fats"? We still recommend that you check the ingredient list for hydrogenated or partially hydrogenated vegetable oils. Ideally, find a way to consume none of these. Keep in mind that the food industry is able to say that the amount of a certain type of fat is "zero" when it's really 0.5 mg.

Step 7: Read the list of ingredients. The ingredients list on food labels can be overwhelming in length, and many of the ingredients listed can be difficult to pronounce or understand! A good rule of thumb is to eat foods made from ingredients that you can recognize and pronounce, and limit the foods you eat that are made from ingredients you can't readily identify. And often, the fewer ingredients the better.

We especially recommend that you try to stay away from artificial sweeteners, flavors, and colors, as well as high-fructose corn syrup, corn syrup, hydrogenated and partially hydrogenated oils, and the wide variety of sugar alcohols (mannitol, sorbitol, maltitol, erythritol, and the like) used in many foods. Artificial sweeteners cause a

Ingredients: Whole wheat flour, dried fruit, wheat bran, high-fructose corn syrup, salt, niacinamide, zinc oxide, reduced iron, pyridoxine hydrochloride (vitamin B_6), riboflavin (vitamin B_2), thiamine hydrochloride (vitamin B_1), folic acid, vitamin A palmitate, vitamin B_{12}, vitamin D, flavoring.

disconnect between what you think you're eating and how your body reacts. The body closely tracks the sensation of "sweet," and whether the sweeteners are real or artificial, smelling sweetness will trigger the body to prepare to eat sweet by producing insulin. So, you release insulin even if the sugar isn't there, and it's the insulin—regardless of sugar source—that can cause problems. It's insulin's job to open the cellular "doors" for glucose and other nutrients. This causes blood glucose to drop, inflammation to increase, and a whole host of other problems to ensue (the reactive-limbic brain starts to drive decision making, and the symptoms you learned about in chapter 1 increase).

Here's a list of carbohydrates that trigger the body to release insulin as if they were sugar sources— starting with what causes the most damage to the body and progressing to what supports the body the most. The bold items are things you should consume very small amounts of.

- **Alcohol**

- **High-fructose corn syrup, corn syrup**

- Fructose, agave syrup

- White sugar, honey, maple syrup, barley syrup

- White bread, pasta, white rice, white potatoes

- Fruit juice

- Dark, thick whole wheat breads

- Whole grains

- Whole fruits

- Vegetables

Fructose, used in "natural sodas" and other foods that make health claims by excluding sugar cane, still impacts the body. Fructose separated from the fruit is metabolized in the body differently from whole-fruit sources because it lacks the fiber and other more complex carbohydrates, which slow the release of the sugar. Fructose as an added sweetener (or in excess) contributes to fatty liver disease, diabetes, and obesity.

Research has shown that there is individual variation in how people react to different carbohydrates. The variation is large enough that it draws into question the utility of the glycemic index, which provides a broad indication of the impact that specific foods will have on blood glucose levels. For example, Kristen has found that her body doesn't register the sugars in potatoes in the same way as it does white rice. Because of this individual variation, we strongly recommend that you experiment with these different foods and monitor your energy level and mental clarity and how soon you feel hungry again after eating. Only then will you have the information you need to make the best decisions for your own body.

ACTION: COMPARE YOUR FAVORITE FOOD LABELS

Practice the steps above to learn more about your favorite packaged foods, such as protein bars, milk substitutes, cereals, pizzas, frozen meals, and others. Remember that this exercise will help you understand how long these foods will keep you fueled and better identify what place they might have in your diet. (For a summary of how to read labels and a worksheet to compare food labels, please refer to http://www.newharbinger.com/46233.)

Food Name:			
Serving size[1]			
Calories			
Total carbs (g)			
Total fiber (g)			
Calculated carbs (g)[2]			
Protein (g)			
Calculated-carb-to-protein ratio			
Category[3] (meal, healthy snack, dessert, sugar rush)			
Real (whole food) ingredients? ☺ ☺ ☹			

Few ingredients? ☺ ☹ ☹			
No sugar alcohols? ☺ ☹ ☹			
Other notes			
Ingredients			

[1] Is the serving size realistic? To make this table a better reference for yourself, make the calculations so your real serving size is reflected.

[2] Calculated carbs = total carbs minus fiber(s).

[3] This identifies the place this food might have in your diet, based on the calculated-carb-to-protein ratio. Our general guidelines are:

- Ratios less than 1:1 to 4:1 = Meal or healthy snack, depending on serving size.
- Ratios 5:1 to 7:1 = Dessert; indulge intentionally and expect to crash one to one and a half hours later unless you eat some protein with it or eat again shortly after.
- Ratios greater than 7:1 = Sugar rush; expect a big high followed by a big low in energy and mental clarity. Choose when to indulge in these foods carefully.

Remember that these ratios assume that you're eating these foods on their own. If you're combining them, calculate the overall calculated-carb-to-protein ratio for the meal or snack.

PUTTING IT ALL TOGETHER

In this chapter we discussed how to read a label to know how the food or meal is likely to make you feel. As you've learned from previous chapters, eating small amounts of protein throughout the day stabilizes blood glucose, the power supply of the brain. Reducing fluctuations in the brain's power supply keeps you in your responsive-cortex brain and prevents your reactive-limbic brain from taking over. This means higher levels of mental clarity and energy, which lead to better decision making and better control over your anxiety levels. Some take-home messages from this chapter are:

- Know what your daily target is for protein. Meals should have 15–25 grams of protein, depending on your weight and (physical) activity level. Experiment to find the amount that supports your energy and mental clarity.

- Know the serving size of the food you're eating and adjust the nutrient contents (from the label) to represent how much of it you actually eat.

- Use the guidance in this chapter to figure out the calculated-carb-to-protein ratio (calculated carbs are total carbohydrates minus fiber) for the foods you eat. This will help you choose foods that will give you the energy you need and keep your anxiety at a manageable level.

- Ignore the "sugars" line on food labels; it doesn't reflect how your body will register the sweetness of a food.

- Limit artificial sweeteners. Don't lie to your body—diet soda, just like regular sodas, can put you at risk for cardiovascular disease, diabetes, and kidney disease.

- Avoid trans fats and hydrogenated and partially hydrogenated fats. Generally, veggie fats are good for you.

There are different calculated-carb-to-protein ratios that can be categorized as meals, desserts, and "sugar rush." Our suggestions:

- Meal or snack ratio: 1–4 calculated carbs to 1 protein will support your energy and reduce your anxiety.

- Dessert ratio: 5–7 calculated carbs to 1 protein should be consumed in smaller quantities and are in the dessert range.

- Sugar rush ratio: Ratios of 8 or more calculated carbs to 1 protein will create a sugar rush; it's okay to indulge in these foods from time to time, but try to make it a conscious decision and avoid overindulging by mindlessly eating these treats.

A meal ratio, even if it's for a snack, should give you the longest time with your responsive-cortex brain engaged. For people who experience generalized anxiety, this often lasts three to four hours; people who exercise a lot might be able to get an additional hour (four to five hours) of being in their responsive-cortex brain. The reason why exercise can help some people stay engaged in their responsive-cortex brains for longer is that exercise temporarily breaks down muscle mass. The amino acids in the protein in muscles enter the blood supply, and can be used as fuel by the liver. People with a history of trauma may need some brain fuel (protein) and a little bit of carbs every two hours. You will have to run your own experiments to know how to optimize your energy and mental clarity.

EXPERIMENT: USING LABELS TO IMPROVE ENERGY AND MENTAL CLARITY

As you start reading food labels, take note of the foods you eat and the ratio of calculated carbs to protein. How long did your energy last? How did the food make you feel?

Date: _____

Is this a meal, a snack, or a treat? _____

Which food did you try? _____

Ratio: _____

How long did your energy last? _____

Is this a food you see yourself adding to your diet for the long term to alleviate anxiety and fatigue?

_____

_____

Date: _____

Is this a meal, a snack, or a treat? _____

Which food did you try? _____

Ratio: _____

How long did your energy last? _____

Is this a food you see yourself adding to your diet for the long term to alleviate anxiety and fatigue?

_____

_____

For many of us, most of our foods come with labels, and it's important to understand what the nutrition information and ingredient lists on those labels mean. But we also recommend that you work to increase the amount of foods in your diet that don't come with labels. Foods without labels that are *real* are *really* good for you when you get a healthy mix of protein, complex carbs, veggies, and healthy fats. Websites like http://www.myfitnesspal.com and http://www.whfoods.org give the nutritional data for "real" foods so you can see how much more nutritional (and tasty) they are.

The Path of Discovery

Kristen was giving a talk at a retirement home where two of the three daily meals were provided, and the residents were responsible for preparing the third in their rooms, which had microwaves and mini refrigerators. She was there to discuss the importance of protein for preventing anxiety, depression, early-morning insomnia, and sarcopenia (muscle loss), which leads to older people falling and injuring themselves. A bright and savvy 75-year-old named Delores asked about limiting sodium to control high blood pressure.

Kristen explained that Delores should experiment with reducing her sodium for two weeks and see if her blood pressure was influenced or not. Not taking a dodge from someone half her age, Delores explained that she did not salt her foods. She did not eat "salty" foods, such as potato chips, but most of her food was no longer freshly produced and came out of a can. She had sat in the kitchen at the residence center as her breakfast and dinner were made, so she knew they had lots of added salt. She wanted to reduce her sodium intake by half. Kristen confirmed that, while Delores was doing her best, people who eat mostly processed foods typically do get too much sodium. Kristen explained that another way to offset your salt intake and prevent hypertension is to eat lots of veggies (5–8 cups per day) and fruits (1–2 servings per day) and to move your body three or four times per week. Of course Kristen's fast-thinking friend wanted to know if they had to be fresh veggies and fruits. Kristen told her that fresh is best, frozen is next, and canned is way better than none at all. And that it's okay to microwave them.

Now this is the best part: Delores said, "I like you, Dr. Allott. I was a science teacher, and the principles I tried to teach my kids were the same as yours: do experiments to find out about the world and yourself, when you hit a barrier find a way around it, and be practical, not perfect—this makes for a more fun and interesting life."

And she was right: those are good principles for life, and this chapter hopefully gave you the information you need to be curious about how you can practice these principles in regard to food. For fatigue and anxiety, it's very important to know how much protein is in the food you're eating and more specifically the calculated-carbohydrate-to-protein ratio. This information will help you predict how you'll feel two to four hours after eating.

CHAPTER SUMMARY

As review, what we learned from the Three-Day Protein Experiment (chapter 4) is that if we want to have more energy and mental clarity, better sleep, and less anxiety and fatigue, we need to eat protein throughout the day to ensure that our brains are getting enough fuel. We also need some carbohydrates, fat, and vegetables that contain fiber and micronutrients, such as B vitamins and minerals. We hope that this chapter helps you understand how to read food labels and that you feel encouraged to do some "eating experiments."

Remember that the brain hates to feel deprived, so we typically recommend that people start by *adding* protein before making other dietary changes, like reducing the number of carbs. When you fuel your body, you'll find that you feel better and will naturally be drawn to making healthier choices around what and how much to eat. The next chapter, "Eating Well for Your Brain in Today's World," provides a number of tools to help with this.

## CHAPTER 6

Eating Well for Your Brain in Today's World

We've now covered the basics: you understand that how you feel is affected by when and what you eat, you have some experience with the Three-Day Protein Experiment, and you know how to interpret labels. What comes next? This chapter provides tools to integrate this information and these new behaviors into your everyday life.

Eating healthy in today's world can be challenging. It's becoming increasingly important to make a plan in advance if you want to take control of what and when you eat and improve how you feel throughout the day. We know meals that contain protein help stabilize blood glucose, helping you stay in your responsive-cortex brain and limiting anxiety and worry. This adds up to you feeling better and having more energy and mental clarity. As a reminder, it's not just the protein—you also need carbohydrates, whole grains, veggies, fruits, and fats to fuel your body and brain to be your best self. This chapter provides tools and tips for purposeful eating.

Benefits of Eating Enough Protein

- ✓ More stable moods
- ✓ More energy
- ✓ Hungry less often
- ✓ Less fatigue, particularly in the afternoons
- ✓ Better sleep
- ✓ Higher metabolism from having higher muscle mass

IDEAS FOR MAINTAINING PROTEIN IN YOUR DIET THROUGHOUT THE DAY

One of the hardest things to do is to decide what to eat. Sometimes having suggestions or sample meals can help you take action. Below is a variety of breakfasts, lunches, and dinners, which are interchangeable, to give you a sense of what protein-rich, balanced meals look like. These meal ideas, like all the tools provided in this chapter, will hopefully encourage the thought, *Oh, I could try that.*

Meal Ideas

BREAKFAST

Goal: *14–20 grams of protein, carbs (bread, pasta, rice, fruit, sweets), veggies (nutrient-rich fiber), and a little fat.*

- 1 cup high-protein plain Greek yogurt (protein) with walnuts, almonds, or cashews (some protein, fiber, fat); raisins, an apple, or ½ a banana (carbs and some fiber)

- Whole eggs: 2–3 scrambled, boiled, or fried (protein, fat); a handful of veggies (nutrient-rich fiber); toast or sweet potato (carbs and some fiber)

- Breakfast burrito with scrambled eggs, tofu, veggie sausage, or refried beans; spinach, onion, and mushrooms; cheese; salsa

- 4 tbsp of nut or seed butter (almond, cashew, or tahini); celery, carrot, or apple

- Make your own protein shake with whey or rice protein powder, dark berries, chocolate powder, and coconut milk or water

- Ready-to-drink protein shake (remember to look at the label for protein, calculated carbs, and real food ingredients)

- Protein bar (remember to look at the label for protein, calculated carbs, and real food ingredients)

A REMINDER ABOUT PROTEIN SHAKES AND BARS

Use the "Compare Your Favorite Food Labels" activity in chapter 5 to find out which shakes and bars work for you. Generally, people do better with a calculated-carb-to-protein ratio of 4:1 or less and real sweeteners (e.g., sugar, honey). Read the ingredients list to check for artificial sweeteners; if it tastes sweeter than the carbs indicate, you might get a larger insulin release and end up in your reactive-limbic brain faster than for products with real sweeteners.

SNACK

Goal: *6–8 grams of protein, ideally with carbs, fiber, and/ or fat.*

- Handful (~¼ cup) of walnuts, almonds, or cashews; maybe include raisins or cranberries (often available in individual bags)

- 2–4 tbsp of nut or seed butter (almond, cashew, or tahini); maybe include carrots, apple, banana, or crackers

- 1–2 hard-boiled eggs, with corn chips

- 1 cup hummus, with chips or veggies

- ½ cup high-protein Greek yogurt; maybe include berries or nuts

- ½ cup cottage cheese, with celery or carrots

- Protein bar

- Jerky (animal- or plant-based); meat sticks

- ½ ready-to-drink protein shake

> **Snacks Act as Lizard Brain Treats—They're Great:**
>
> 1. Between meals
> 2. Between different activities, such as leaving work or school to go home
> 3. Before big emotional challenges
> 4. To give to kids (or adults) before they melt down

LUNCH

Goal: *20 grams of protein, 1–2 cups of veggies (nutrient-rich fiber), carbs (bread, pasta, rice, fruit, sweets), and fat.*

- Animal- or plant-based protein on a salad, burrito, wrap, or sandwich; over rice or pasta; or in soup

- 1 cup high-protein Greek yogurt with walnuts, almonds, or cashews; dried dark berries

- Egg salad on toast with a bed of salad greens

- Three-bean or lentil salad with quinoa

SNACK

Goal: *6–8 grams of protein, ideally with carbs, fiber, and/or fat.*

- Same as previous snack examples

DINNER

Goal: *20 grams of protein, 1–2 cups of veggies (nutrient-rich fiber), carbohydrates (bread, pasta, rice, fruit, sweets), and fat*

- Animal- or plant-based protein on a salad, burrito, wrap, or sandwich, or over rice or pasta

- A can of soup with added animal- or plant-based protein and a quick salad of canned artichoke hearts with salad dressing

- Quinoa pasta with animal- or plant-based protein, red sauce, and veggies; and a side salad

- Animal- or plant-based protein chili, with roasted veggies (sweet potato, parsnip, carrots, beets, and Brussels sprouts)

- Beans on quinoa with cooked, previously frozen broccoli and 1 tbsp of butter

- Animal- or plant-based protein stir-fry with veggies on quinoa or brown rice

- Quesadilla with animal- or plant-based protein, spinach or sautéed mushrooms, onions, and cheddar cheese

Now that you have some ideas, or a possible starter menu, the next tool will help you build meals and snacks on your own.

TAKE THE OVERWHELM OUT OF FIGURING OUT WHAT TO EAT

We make so many decisions throughout each day. Sometimes we're too tired or overwhelmed, or just lack interest in deciding what to eat. But we still need to feed ourselves healthy food if we want to be at our best. Having a list of go-to foods pinned to the fridge can be helpful when making decisions about what to eat feels difficult. Below are some ideas to get you started.

Mix and Match Food Choices and Preparation Styles

PROTEIN		VEGGIES	
Choices	Preparation	Choices	Preparation
ANIMAL PROTEIN	**ANIMAL PROTEIN**	**LEAFY GREENS***	Baked
Chicken	Baked	Lettuces, mesclun mix	Dipped
Turkey	Broiled	Broccoli	Fermented/pickled
Beef	Fried	Spinach	Grilled
Lamb	Grilled	Kale, chard, collards	In salad
Pork	Instant Pot	Bok choy	Instant Pot
Fish, tuna, shellfish	Microwaved	Cabbage (green, red)	Microwaved
Ground meat (beef,	Poached	Brussels sprouts	Raw and naked (finger
turkey, pork)	Slow cooked		food)
Sausage (chicken, pork,		**OTHER VEGGIES***	Sautéed
turkey)		Garlic	Slow cooked
Bacon (pork, turkey)		Onions	Steamed
Healthy sandwich meat		Celery	Stuffed and baked
		Tomatoes	
LEGUMES*	**LEGUMES**	Mushrooms	
Tofu	Baked	Cucumber	
Tempeh	Boiled	Carrots	
Lentils	Fried	String beans	
Beans	Grilled	Bell peppers	
Plant-based protein	Instant Pot	Zucchini	
burgers	Microwaved	Summer squash	
	Slow cooked	Peas	
		Edamame	
		Eggplant	

PROTEIN		CARBS	
Choices	Preparation	Choices	Preparation
OTHER PROTEIN SOURCES	**OTHER PROTEIN SOURCES**	Bread, muffins	Baked
Egg	As part of hot cereal	Pancakes, waffles	Boiled
Cottage cheese	Boiled (hard, soft)	Tortillas	Broiled
Nuts, seeds	Fried in salads	Oatmeal,* grits*	Fried
Nut butters	In shakes/smoothies	High fiber/high protein	Grilled
Soy cheese, soy yogurt	Microwaved	cereals*	In hot or cold salads
Greek yogurt	Poached	Potatoes (all colors)	Instant Pot
Protein powders (whey,	Scrambles, frittatas	Rice (brown,* white)	Mashed
rice, soy)	With fruit	Sweet potatoes*	Microwaved
Quinoa*		Winter squashes*	Slow cooked
Barley*		Fruits*	Toasted

SNACKS/TREATS	FATS	RARE INDULGENCES
Dark chocolate	Butter	*Good as a delight, but can be hard on the*
Cottage Cheese	Oils (olive, sesame seed,	*body, so best to have in small quantities:*
Apples*	safflower, coconut)	
Banana* with nut butter	Cheese	Ice cream, cakes, candy, doughnuts, etc.
Protein bars	Avocado	
Carrots* and hummus	Nuts,* nut butters	*All count as carbs.*
Nuts,* nut butters		

*　Fiber sources

Circle the ones you like and add favorites that aren't listed. Remember to mix and match from the categories: protein, carbs, fiber, and fat.

If the above table is overwhelming or we missed your favorites, create your own version from this blank form (both charts are available for download at http://www.newharbinger.com/46233).

Making sure the food you enjoy is in the house will give you ready options to work with.

Tips for Prepping Meals

The following suggestions are some ways to make meal preparation easier. Having food prepared in advance can ease your worry about managing your anxiety.

Healthy foods can be delivered to your home in all sorts of ways, including CSAs (community-supported agriculture farms/gardens), grocery delivery, restaurant delivery, and meal delivery of fully prepared or pre-prepped and measured meals. These come in all food preferences and quantity of meals.

There are also some places where you can go and do the prep yourself with all ingredients made available, and you leave with fridge- and freezer-ready complete meals.

- If you have more time to cook over the weekend, make extra and freeze it. If you know you're going to have a long day, take the meal out in the morning, and then all you have to do is heat it up when you get home.

- Precook meats. For example, chicken, turkey, and pork sausages are about 3 oz. each (21 g protein) and can be added to leftovers, salads, a can of soup, a burrito, stir-fry, or prepared veggies picked up at a deli.

- Experiment with slow cookers. You can put everything in the cooker the night before and stash it in the fridge. Turn it on in the morning and come home to a dinner that's ready to eat!

  - Slow cookers are great for making yummy meats. It's easy to find recipes on the internet; "pulled" chicken and pork are awesome on everything!

  - Slow cookers are great for veggies. Try squash, sweet potatoes, beets, carrots, onions, or garlic. Just put them in on low and walk away for six to eight hours. Sometimes they are perfect; sometimes they need a little more cooking. Even if occasionally overcooked, they're edible. The big advantage is that it's easy and the veggies are ready to eat!

PROTEIN		VEGGIES	
Choices	Preparation	Choices	Preparation
ANIMAL PROTEIN	ANIMAL PROTEIN	LEAFY GREENS*	
		OTHER VEGGIES*	
LEGUMES*	LEGUMES		
OTHER PROTEIN SOURCES	OTHER PROTEIN SOURCES		

CARBS*	
Choices	Preparation

SNACKS/TREATS	FATS	RARE INDULGENCES
		Good as a delight, but can be hard on the body, so best to have in small quantities: *All count as carbs.*

*   Fiber sources

There are many excellent websites and cookbooks tailored to different food preferences that give tips on how to prepare foods; we provide links to some of these as well as more ideas on using food to maintain energy and mental clarity amid a busy life at http://www.kristenallott.com/blog.

Eating Well at Work

Maintaining energy and mental clarity and reducing anxiety do take some planning, particularly for meals at work. Most people, when they do it, report feeling better. Here are some suggestions to make this possible.

- Make extra dinner, or cook enough over the weekend to have leftovers for a few lunches.

- Get the right containers—for example, glass containers that can easily be microwaved—and a fun lunch bag. Having something to bring food to work in is key. Getting something that you like the look and functionality of will make it more enjoyable to use.

- Make a list of restaurants, delis, and corner shops near where you work. Get or print out menus and circle the healthy choices that are in line with your dietary goals. Having these preselected helps reduce "impulse ordering."

- Keep backup emergency snacks in a drawer: protein bars with enough protein so they can be meal replacements in a pinch, a jar of nut butter, bags of nuts and dried fruit, and dark chocolate bars are convenient to store at work.

As you begin working to implement the guidance in this chapter and the previous ones in your day-to-day life, remember that the three-day experiment you did was based on 68–76 grams of protein a day. This may be a little more or less than what you need for your body weight. To reduce anxiety and worry, and improve energy and mental clarity, make sure that you're thinking about your daily protein target as you explore meal ideas or build meal plans. To help with this, use the next tool to create a plan for meals when you're busy.

WHAT IS YOUR EMERGENCY FOOD PLAN?

There are busy days, and there are terrible-horrible-no-good days. On the worst of days, most of us still manage to brush our teeth because it's hardwired into the brain. However, eating in a way that supports our energy and mental clarity is one of the easiest things to drop. Having a written emergency food plan to take the thought out of how and what to feed yourself will help you be at your best on these very challenging days. If you preplan for these days, there is a greater possibility that you'll fuel your brain when you need it most. It's important to build flexibility into the plan. For example: have healthy, quick meal options at home; identify places you can get ready-made food (restaurants, grocery stores, takeout), and include menus and numbers for meal delivery options.

Here are some ideas:

- Mac and cheese with frozen peas and chicken or skipjack tuna

- Healthy frozen meals

- Ramen soup package with an egg or precooked animal- or plant-based protein

- Salad bar with a lot of variety at a restaurant or grocery store

- List the names of stores or restaurants on your frequently traveled paths

- Circle healthy choices on the menus of your favorite delivery options

Use the table below as a template for creating your own emergency food plan. Having three ideas for each meal will help you stay on track. Be sure to check that each meal has protein, carbs, fiber, and fat. There are no rules against eating dinner for breakfast and breakfast for dinner! The goal is to have some ideas that you don't have to think too much about. Remember: eating sets you up for having the energy and mental clarity you need to deal with the business of the day and will keep your anxiety and worry physiologically in check.

Use the table below as a template for creating your own emergency food plan.

Breakfast	Lunch	Dinner
1.	1.	1.
2.	2.	2.
3.	3.	3.

WHAT ARE YOUR TREATS?

As you start to organize your diet to support energy and mental clarity, it may be tempting to try to cut out all treats. Our experience is that this just leads to binge-eating. To avoid this, it can be helpful to identify specific foods that you're not willing to give up. Note that we haven't taken away your favorite foods; we've mostly just added protein. With more protein, hopefully you're experiencing fewer sugar cravings. Use the space below to get a clearer picture of your favorite treats.

What foods are you not willing to remove from your diet at this time?

What are some healthier treats that work for you most of the time? These are treats that don't crash your energy or wipe you out later in the day.

What are the treats that can get you in trouble? Can you think of any substitutes that would still satisfy your craving but might work a little bit better for you and that you can commit to swapping in as consistently as you can?

WHY YOU BINGE ON SUGAR AFTER A BAD DAY

As an important side note, have you ever noticed that when you have had a really bad day, you crave food that has sugar? There are different reasons why we crave sugar:

- Your brain needs more glucose so you can be at your best.

- Your brain is trying to prevent the adrenaline from being released.

- When we consume food high in carbohydrates (candy, cookies, cake, chips, and ice cream, to name the common ones), our brains make the neurotransmitter serotonin. Serotonin tells our brains that "Everything is okay." However, it takes about twenty minutes after eating for you to get that signal.

If this sounds familiar, here's an easy experiment to try:

1. What's your go-to treat after a bad day? _____

2. How much of it do you typically eat? _____

3. What amount would feel more comfortable as a single serving? _____

4. The next time you have that craving, try serving yourself a single serving and waiting twenty minutes. Remember, the promise you can make to yourself is that you can have more if you still want it after the twenty minutes.

5. If you've tried the experiment, take some time to write about how it went. If you eat more after the twenty minutes is up, that's okay! Try to be curious about yourself; you're just collecting data. The idea is that if you wait twenty minutes, you might get the signal that "Everything is okay," and you might not eat more than a serving.

Since Natasha learned that it took twenty minutes for her brain to give her the signal, "Everything is okay, and my brain is refueled," she still goes for the treats after a bad day. However, instead of sitting down with a pint of ice cream, she now serves herself two scoops in a bowl. She tells herself that she can have more, but not until she waits twenty minutes. More often than not, the craving is gone by then. This stopped her from adding devouring an entire pint of ice cream to the list of why it was a bad day—she wasn't left with the physical and emotional aftereffects of too much ice cream.

SHIFT YOUR ATTENTION

Food is a major form of entertainment. Unfortunately, this often means mindless eating of nonnutritious calories. It's often easier to break this habit by finding replacements instead of trying to "just stop." Here are a few things to try:

- Change what you mindlessly eat. Try to add foods high in protein while decreasing the amount of your "mouth entertainment items."

- Put your snack in a small bowl. Setting out a specific portion helps prevent eating a whole bag of something or an entire pint of ice cream. If you still want more when you've finished it, wait twenty minutes before getting more so that your brain has time to catch up with the food you just ate.

- Replace eating with other forms of entertainment. When do you use food as entertainment? Understanding your patterns will help you think of ways to replace food with other, healthier activities, such as drawing, coloring, knitting, developing a hobby, or playing a musical instrument.

CHAPTER SUMMARY

Chapters 3 through 6 focused on understanding the impact that food has on your physiology; hopefully, you now have new tools to reduce anxiety, worry, and fatigue. While food is an important factor, sleep and movement are also determinants of your power supply. The next chapter focuses on the first of these, looking at how sleep can recharge your brain and power supply.

Part III

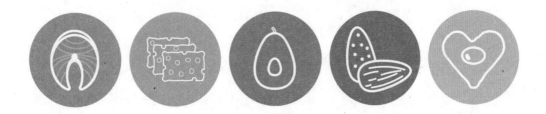

More Experiments to Improve Energy and Reduce Anxiety

## CHAPTER 7

Fueling Your Brain for Better Sleep

We know that sleep is essential for clear thinking and provides vibrant energy that allows us to engage in the challenges and passions of our lives. But there are many things that can disturb sleep, from early-morning waking to nightmares and night terrors. Medications that override these challenges don't provide restful sleep and often leave people drowsy in the morning. Many anxiety and fatigue symptoms around sleep can be addressed through protein solutions and improved sleep rituals. In this chapter, you'll get to see Luca practice some of these new tools.

In this chapter, we explain how supporting glucose control and creating rituals around sleep can help correct some dysfunctional sleep patterns, including:

- Being awake for two hours in the middle of the night

- Nightmares

- PTSD nightmares and night terrors

- Waking up with anxiety

- Having a hard time waking up

- Not being hungry in the morning

- Afternoon fatigue

It's helpful to start with an understanding of why we need sleep and how much sleep we need. Then, we'll provide a checklist for behaviors that support good sleep, address glucose regulation issues that disrupt sleep, and explore rituals for improving sleep to reduce fatigue and anxiety.

WHY WE NEED SLEEP

Sleep is not a passive activity for our bodies or brains. If we think back to the four quadrants of self presented in the introduction—the body, the brain, relationships, and the mind—the mind may be offline while we're sleeping and our relationships not consciously active, but the body and brain are busy preparing for the next day. During sleep we synthesize neurotransmitters (dopamine and serotonin) that we'll use during the next day, our memories consolidate themselves and keep our sense of the past coherent, and our hormonal systems reset themselves, just to name a few important sleep-time activities. We could go on, as the list of the many things that the body and brain do while we are "out for the night" is lengthy. We often equate it to a large office building. If people don't come in during the night to take out the trash, restock the paper, and vacuum the floor, the office won't run as efficiently the next day. Sleep is an important activity if we want to increase our resilience and decrease our anxiety and fatigue.

Studies are clear that if we're sleep deprived, we'll have increased:

- Symptoms of psychiatric conditions such as anxiety, depression, ADHD, and bipolar

- Difficulty learning and remembering new material (memories won't be consolidated)

- Fatigue

- Inflammation (which can present as symptoms of pain, increased blood pressure, and weight gain)

Additionally, important brain structures, such as the hippocampus, will have less new cell creation, which can impair learning and memory. When we get enough sleep, we're helping increase the brain's ability to learn and rewire itself (neuroplasticity).

HOW MUCH SLEEP IS ENOUGH?

For people over 18 years old, getting between seven and nine hours of sleep can help optimize how we experience and engage in our lives. Either side of that range has been shown to negatively affect cognitive performance, such as effective reasoning, problem solving, and communication. What's more, studies consistently show that too little sleep and too much sleep can have similar negative effects on our physical and mental health.

Chronic undersleeping is a common problem for those suffering with anxiety and fatigue. In studies where people are getting six hours of sleep for four nights, instead of their regular eight hours, people's internal experience is that they are having cognitive deficits for the first two days. After that, they believe that they have adjusted and are doing fine. In fact, they haven't recovered their prior cognitive skills. It's difficult for a brain that isn't functioning well to determine if it's functioning well. Plus, there's a survival mechanism that kicks in when there is too much stress (emotional, physical, mental). At first the brain–body says, "Too much!" But if we don't address the stressor, our minds adjust to the "new normal," we start to think that everything is okay, and the body starts to cope with what is happening. But this doesn't mean that it's optimal or our best. For the short term—say, when we're at a crucial time in school or have a new baby in the house—we can cope with lack of sleep. However, if we don't take time to recover, both physical and mental health challenges can increase.

Consistently undersleeping can increase the risk of conditions associated with inflammation, such as anxiety, depression, bipolar disorder, diabetes, cardiovascular disease, weight gain, some cancers, and dementia, to name a few. Additionally, not getting enough sleep over decades can shorten your life. If you're a poor sleeper, improving sleep is a worthy goal to move toward! In this chapter, we're going to provide some tools to experiment with to see if you can change your sleep patterns. Improved sleep will increase your body's power supply to your brain and decrease your anxiety and fatigue.

There are some common patterns that people have that disrupt their sleep. We'll discuss these patterns and give you tools to improve falling asleep, staying asleep, and waking up refreshed in the mornings. But first, let's cover the basics.

> ### Recommended Hours of Sleep
>
> - Older adults (65+): 7–8 hours
> - Adults (26–64): 7–9 hours
> - Younger adults (18–25): 7–9 hours
> - Teenagers (14–17): 8–10 hours
> - School-age children (6–13): 9–11 hours
> - Preschoolers (3–5): 10–13 hours
> - Toddlers (1–2 years): 11–14 hours
> - Infants (4–11 months): 12–15 hours
> - Newborns (0–3 months): 14–17 hours
>
> *From the National Sleep Foundation, http://www.sleepfoundation.org.*

COMMON SLEEP CHALLENGES

If your sleep is being interrupted by anxiety or anxiety-like symptoms, such as a racing mind, nightmares, or waking up anxious, we'll give you protein solutions to address these and more. Not getting enough sleep or sleeping poorly can contribute to fatigue, worry, and anxiety throughout the day. To improve both the quantity and quality of your sleep, there are some important routines or rituals that you can experiment with that can improve your power supply, thereby decreasing fatigue, worry, and anxiety. In this chapter we'll cover:

- Protein solutions for the following sleep-related challenges:
  - Early-morning waking
  - Nightmares
  - PTSD nightmares and night terrors
  - Waking up with anxiety
  - Oversleeping, not being functional in the morning
  - Not being hungry for breakfast
  - Afternoon fatigue
- Other important rituals that support healthy sleep:
  - Establishing routines
  - Solutions for snoring
  - Feeling safe when sleeping

PROTEIN SOLUTIONS FOR HEALTHY SLEEP

While sleep challenges manifest themselves in different ways for different people, one of the driving factors for all of them is the same: insufficient fuel supply for the brain. Back in chapter 3, we learned how fueling the body and brain can impact mood. It can also impact sleep and contribute to all of the issues listed above.

But first, let's talk about what typically happens at night: We eat our last meal. It could be large or small. It could be right before bed or hours before bed. Many people eat a lot of refined carbohydrates in this meal (bread, pasta, pizza, rice, potatoes, dessert, and/or alcohol). This causes a release of insulin to move the glucose—carbohydrates broken down into glucose in your digestive tract—from your bloodstream into your cells. We may not get an adrenaline release two to three hours after eating dinner because we're typically not thinking as much or as hard in the evenings. So, we have fuel to go to sleep.

As we discussed earlier, the brain is super busy while we sleep. Our brains need energy to be able to prepare for the next day. Because you're sleeping—and not eating—your brain and body can become low in fuel. This causes an adrenaline release, which initiates fuel production by the liver. While this addresses the immediate need for fuel, adrenaline at night causes many problematic sleep patterns. We discuss below some sleep disturbances that might be happening to you.

Awake for two hours. An adrenaline release can wake you up for around two hours in the middle of the night with what we call a "3:00 a.m. committee meeting." This two-hour meeting can occur at other times than 3:00 a.m.; however, it often occurs at this time for people who go to bed around 10:00 p.m. This is when your brain races in the middle of the night, reviewing what someone said, what you could have said, what you should or should not do, and all the possible problems that might happen. This is caused by the adrenaline in your body waking you and your stressed-out brain and reminding you of everything that is going on—usually in a fairly critical internal voice that would make anyone anxious. And the result is that you lose two hours of precious sleep—setting you up for more stress later on.

Nightmares. Sometimes you don't wake up with the adrenaline release, but your brain will put together a story to justify all the adrenaline. This is your basic nightmare: running, falling, screaming, or just disturbing dreams.

PTSD nightmares and night terrors. If you have a history that includes seeing or experiencing violence, physical, verbal, or sexual abuse, instability, or being overwhelmed, your brain might pull forward those events or mental states and recall them as you sleep because your brain is running out of fuel as you sleep. This can create a cycle in which you want to avoid sleep because you don't want to revisit the past. But the lack of sleep makes it harder to contain the past, so during the day you may have a higher level of anxiety as well as increased fatigue from not getting restful sleep.

Waking up with anxiety. You may wake up with anxiety or irritation for no particular reason. Physiologically, adrenaline has likely been released to make fuel for your brain. However, the adrenaline has also moved you into your reactive-limbic system, which approaches the present moment with fear, anger, agitation, or numbness. Waking up anxious or stressed is a challenging way to start the day. Here, also, you may not want to eat because of all the adrenaline in your system.

Not hungry for breakfast. You may also tend to wake up not hungry when adrenaline is on board. It's your body's natural tendency not to be hungry when you're running from a bear or other primal threat. Additionally, when there is adrenaline in your system, less blood goes to your digestive system, which means that the digestive system is not prepared to receive food.

Hard to wake up in the morning. You may also have a hard time waking up. Some people sleep through alarms and oversleep by hours, getting 10 to 12 hours of sleep, and still wake up feeling fatigued. This is also a glucose supply problem. You may be thinking that you don't *want* adrenaline, but remember that fueling your body and brain takes precedence, and adrenaline is the "call button." For some people, the call button no longer works for a variety of reasons: not enough adrenaline is released to make enough glucose to fuel your brain, and your glucose level continues to decline, causing you to struggle with waking. You're in a bad state when you do wake up: disoriented or lacking motivation to start your day. You need to get glucose to your brain quickly in order to function.

Fatigue in the afternoon or eight hours after waking. Not sleeping well and not eating breakfast set you up to be tired around 4:00 to 5:00 p.m. on a typical workday, or eight to ten hours after waking.

CHECKLIST FOR GOOD SLEEP

Below is a list of behaviors that have been shown to help most people sleep better. You can use this list to get ideas for supporting your current habits or to help you when you're traveling or sleeping somewhere new. If you're not getting good sleep, look over this list and consider what action(s) you might experiment with. For now, this is just to get you thinking about changes that might be possible for you; we'll get into specific suggestions for experiments later in the chapter.

Action	I do this.	I'll try this.
Go to bed about the same time most nights (+/– one hour).		
Get up about the same time most mornings (+/– one hour).		
Take a hot bath or shower before bed.		
Sleep in a dark room.		
Sleep in a quiet room.		
Sleep in a room that is cool in temperature.		
Sleep in a room without screens (no electronic devices, TVs, and so forth).		
Use an alarm clock instead of a cell phone.		
Use the bed only for sleep and sex.		
Don't look at screens for at least 30 minutes before bed.		

Action	I do this.	I'll try this.
Limit caffeine and chocolate after 2:00 p.m.		
Don't drink alcohol within four hours before bed.		
Get regular exercise (see chapter 8).		

It's also important to pay attention to your individual needs. Have you noticed any conditions that help you sleep? Or activities that wind you up at night?

PROTEIN EXPERIMENTS FOR HEALTHY SLEEP

The following experiments address the physiological disruptions of sleep. We encourage you to try the ones that address your most common sleep issues. Many of them are complementary, so you can also read through all of them and use them together. *Note: It can take 10 to 14 days to see the impact of experiments for improving sleep.* Using your Snapshot of Anxiety Assessment before and after an experiment will help you recognize how sleeping better reduces anxiety, worry, and fatigue.

Fuel Your Brain Before Sleep

People who experience sleep disturbances in the middle of the night or don't wake up feeling refreshed can experiment with fueling their brains before bed because these disruptions might be caused by the brain running out of fuel while you sleep. These disturbances might include:

☐ The 3:00 a.m. "committee meeting"

☐ Nightmares

- ☐ PTSD night terrors

- ☐ Waking with anxiety, irritation, agitation, disorientation, or numbness

- ☐ Waking up not hungry

- ☐ Not being able to wake up.

Check off the ones you're struggling with.

Experiment with fueling your brain before sleep. Try adding a protein snack (7–10 grams) within thirty minutes before going to bed. This could be a couple slices of turkey, a quarter cup of cottage cheese or Greek yogurt, or a quarter cup of nuts. See the protein chart in chapter 4 for more ideas.

Some people have been told that they shouldn't eat before they go to bed. It's true that eating a large meal before bed isn't conducive to good sleep or health. However, what we're suggesting is to eat a small amount of protein in order to improve your sleep, which in turn supports your health and well-being.

But do make sure it's protein that you're eating. If you have a lot of high-carbohydrate foods (sweets, chips, alcohol) before bed or drink caffeine after 2:00 p.m., this is likely to make it harder to fall asleep or could wake you after you've fallen asleep. Ideally, it's better to decrease intake of these foods and drinks in the hours before you go to bed.

Have a Lizard Brain Treat

Eating protein before you go to bed is prevention. Lizard Brain Treats—which, as you'll recall from chapter 3, are treats of about 6 to 8 grams of protein, for example, a quarter cup of nuts, plus a quarter cup of fruit juice—address sleep challenges in the moment. If you experience sleep disturbances in the middle of the night—whether it's the 3:00 a.m. committee meeting, nightmares, or night terrors—fueling your brain as soon as you wake up can help you go back to sleep faster. If you remember the physiology, the juice provides the quick fuel, which turns off the body's call for fuel (through adrenaline) and will help you fall back asleep faster. The nuts provide the protein (and some fat and fiber too!), which is the longer-lasting fuel that will prevent another adrenaline release and help you stay asleep longer.

Experiment with Lizard Brain Treats

For this experiment, put your Lizard Brain Treat on your bed stand for easy access.

- If you have a 3:00 a.m. committee meeting, eat your Lizard Brain Treat upon waking, and you'll likely go back to sleep within 30 minutes.

- If you have nightmares or PTSD night terrors, and if you wake to pee before you commonly have nightmares, eat the Lizard Brain Treat to prevent the nightmare. If you wake from a nightmare, eat the Lizard Brain Treat to recover from the nightmare.

Use the space below to record the results as you try this experiment.

Prioritizing Breakfast

This experiment is for you if you:

- ☐ Wake with anxiety, irritation, agitation, disorientation, or numbness

- ☐ Wake up not hungry

- ☐ Have afternoon fatigue

- ☐ Struggle to wake up

If you wake up and aren't hungry for breakfast, have a hard time functioning, or feel numb or detached, you likely already have adrenaline in your system. You may not feel hungry, but your brain and body need fuel! Starting with a quarter cup of juice (or a small juice box) shortly after waking will shift your body out of survival mode, which will allow your digestive system to reengage. This will make it easier to eat a balanced breakfast (protein, healthy carbs, healthy fat, and fiber) within 20 to 30 minutes.

What we do in the morning may seem like a long way from what we experience eight hours later. But the truth is that breakfast is really important to having a good day and finishing the day with energy. And when we don't eat within an hour after waking, we burn through our supplies of fuel and hormones. But when we eat a balanced breakfast in the morning within an hour of waking, we tend to have better moods in the morning, crave less sugar later in the day, have more sustained energy throughout the day, and most importantly, tend not to crash around 4:00 or 5:00 p.m.

Experiments in Prioritizing Breakfast

1. If you wake with anxiety, irritation, agitation, disorientation, or numbness, or are not hungry, immediately get a quick fuel into your system to help your brain become oriented to the day. Put a quarter cup of juice (or a small juice box), or other quick fuel, on your nightstand and drink it immediately upon waking. This will make it easier to be hungry for a balanced breakfast within an hour.

2. If you have afternoon fatigue, prioritize eating a balanced breakfast within an hour of waking, which will prevent you from burning through your glucose and hormones, causing you to crash in the late afternoon. Chapter 6 provides tools to help you get this done.

3. If you struggle to wake up and you're spending more than 10 hours in bed, put a quarter cup of juice (or a small juice box) and a protein bar on your bed stand and eat it immediately upon waking. The protein bar should have a calculated-carb-to-protein ratio between 2-to-1 and 4-to-1, with at least 9 grams of protein (see chapter 5 for more information on calculated carbs). This will get a more robust amount of fuel into your system faster. This may need to be done daily, ideally at the same time, for at least 10 days before you may begin to have an easier time waking up. Additionally, be sure to eat protein before going to bed.

4. To build on the benefits of breakfast, do the Three-Day Protein Experiment in addition to eating breakfast within an hour of waking (see chapter 4). This will help stabilize your moods throughout the day, increase energy, decrease sugar cravings, and set you up for better sleep.

Use the space below to jot down results of your experiments to improve sleep over the next 10 to 14 days.

Beyond fuel disturbances disrupting sleep, there are a number of other modern-day challenges, like stress and difficulty with scheduling, that keep us from refreshing our power supply at night. If you're struggling with these, having particular bedtime rituals can help.

RITUALS THAT IMPROVE SLEEP AND REDUCE FATIGUE AND ANXIETY

In this section, we'll talk about behaviors that can improve sleep, thereby reducing fatigue and anxiety.

Establishing a Sleep Routine

Having a routine is the best way to train your brain and body to fall asleep. The efficiency of our bodies is governed by circadian clocks. These cellular clocks are looking for behaviors to occur about the same time in the day. One of the systems governed heavily by our routines is our hormone system. The hormone system is the messenger system from the brain to the rest of the body. The brain's messages to the cells include all sorts of information: when to wake up, when to sleep, when to digest food, when to create energy, when to menstruate. When these routines are disrupted, it signals to the body that it's not safe. This can create fatigue and physical health problems, such as obesity and diabetes, as well as mental health problems. When someone is going to sleep at widely varying times, for example sometimes at 8:00 p.m. and sometimes at 2:00 a.m., it's very hard to improve their mental health functioning because the body is spending so much time orienting itself and trying to predict when food and sleep will arrive. When we don't have a rhythm to our day, by eating and sleeping at about the same time, we use our power supplies to deal with the variations, which can exhaust us and make it harder to have the energy to implement strategies to maintain a lower level of anxiety.

The best solution to this problem is to have a set time for going to bed and a set time for waking—and ideally, getting the optimal seven to nine hours of sleep. But having a consistent sleep routine will help too. Different people have different ways of signaling to their bodies that it's time to sleep. What do you do before you go to bed? Do you have a routine? Are you interested in trying to establish one?

Experiment with Establishing a Sleep Routine

Decide when you want to consistently be in bed and when you want to get up, and then try some of the following to help you follow through with this intention:

- Shower or bathe

- Drink a cup of tea

- Meditate or pray

- Journal or write three things that you are grateful for

- Read a book

- Use an essential oil, such as lavender or rose, in your bedroom or on your pillow.

Use the space below to write down when you ideally want to be in bed, when you want to wake up, and what ritual(s) you're going to experiment with to signal to your body that it's time for bed. Keep notes on any changes you experience.

Screen-Free Time Before Bed

One of the most common reasons that people miss the time that they want to go to sleep is that they're in front of a screen. You might be reading an electronic book, watching a movie, surfing the web or social media, or responding to email. All of these will wake you up or drive you to do just one more thing. So be sure to turn off the screen, whether it's your phone, tablet, computer, or TV, 30 to 60 minutes before bedtime. If you have screens in your bedroom, know that many people benefit from removing them from the bedroom altogether. This may require you to get an alarm clock to wake you up in the morning (other than the one on your phone—you remember, one of those old-fashioned things you plug into the wall?). By eliminating screens from the bedroom, you are also establishing another important routine: that your bed is for sleep and sex only. Using your bed for something other than sleep or sex wires into your brain that it doesn't need to go to sleep in that environment.

Often people feel a bit at a loss when they turn off their screens, not being able to think of what else to do. What did you enjoy doing as a kid, or what do you want to practice? This screen-free time is you-time. When you're on a screen, your attention is somewhere else. When you do these other activities, which are interesting but not too stimulating, they can become part of your ritual of going to bed.

When you first try to separate from screens before bed, your brain will tell you that you need to go back to your screen, and this is normal—but if you can resist for at least two weeks, you'll feel the benefits of sleeping better, being less anxious upon waking, and less fatigued throughout the day.

If you're not willing to remove screens from the bedroom, there are still experiments you can try. For instance, try noticing the impact of crime or other high-adrenaline shows or books on your sleep versus themes that are calmer. Remember: your brain encodes the last emotional content of the day. What do you want that to be?

Experiments for Screen-Free Time

1. Decide what time (30–60 minutes before bed) you will turn off your screens. _____

2. Make a list of alternative activities that you want to do during this time, that are about *you* (not a list of "shoulds"). Here is a short list of ideas: draw, color, sing, play an instrument, knit, write, play cards or a board game, do light yoga or stretch, take a bath, listen to music, call a friend or family member, or start or refresh a hobby.

3. Use this time to work on establishing a bedtime routine (see above).

4. Get an alarm clock to use instead of using your phone or device.

Do this consistently for two weeks, and feel the benefits. Come back to this page and note if fatigue and anxiety have improved.

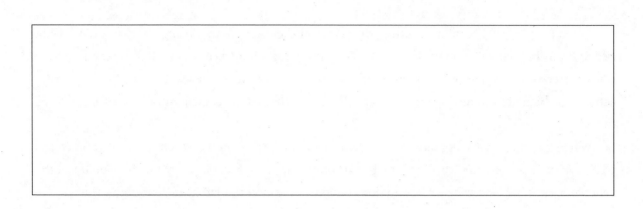

Pay Attention to Your Sleep Clock

Know your sleep-clock pattern. Kristen isn't a good sleeper. Because of this, she's had to make a study of all the tricks to improve her sleep; otherwise, her dyslexic brain dominates her life. She noticed that sometimes she could just fall asleep and other times she would lie awake, tossing and turning. Going to bed early didn't help because it still took her until 11:00 p.m. to fall asleep. Occasionally, Kristen was able to get to bed and fall asleep at 9:30 p.m., but on most nights, she had a hard time getting to bed before 10:00, and then she'd just lie awake until 11:00. Somewhere along the way, Kristen learned about what she describes as *sleep clocks*.

In the evenings, the body starts to prepare for sleep: we get a wave of hormones that will momentarily make us sleepy. This lasts for just five or ten minutes, and then for most people, it kicks in again somewhere between an hour to an hour and a half later. While some people start feeling this sensation as early as 6:00 p.m., Kristen starts to feel sleepy at 8:00; she feels pretty tired, but about ten minutes later, she's just fine until around 9:30. If her head is on the pillow and she turns out the lights at 9:30 p.m., she can quickly fall asleep. Even though she knows this, she often "blows it" by reading a book. By 9:45 p.m., she's tired but not able to fall asleep. When this happens, she might read a bit more or sometimes she just lies there and rests. Knowing that sleep will come at 11:00 p.m. helps her not be anxious about not falling asleep—she's learned the rhythm of her body. What's important is that she doesn't do something overstimulating, such as watching shows about investigating murders, responding to email, or even floating through social media. While not everyone has the experience of a sleep clock, it can be really helpful to try to tune in to your body and learn its more subtle patterns. These can cue you in to the best times to give your body what it needs.

Experiments in following your sleep clock. Observe for a couple of days when your waves of sleepiness show up. Try to be in bed, with your head on the pillow, ready for sleep when you expect one of the waves to arrive. Was it easier to go to sleep?

Sleep-Clock Times:

1st bell: _____

2nd bell: _____

3rd bell: _____

When did you put your head on your pillow? _____

Were you able to fall asleep more easily? _____

Did you wake feeling well rested? _____

Snoring Can Disrupt Your Power Supply, Causing Anxiety and Fatigue

If you are fatigued and a snorer, you can try a couple of things that most people are reluctant to try, but after they do try them and feel better, they continue the new behaviors. The easiest option is to try using nasal strips. These are pieces of tape (available at drugstores or major grocery chains) that you stick on your nose at night. They keep your nasal passages a little more open. This can reduce the effort to breathe, and also the sound. This might help you as well as your bed partner. Either way, if you think snoring may be preventing you from getting a good night's sleep, we encourage you to give nasal strips a try. Many people notice that they wake up more easily and feel ready to get up in the morning.

The second experiment that snorers with fatigue can try is getting a sleep apnea assessment at a sleep clinic. Some snorers intermittently stop breathing on and off throughout the night. When breathing patterns are disrupted, there is less oxygen going to your body and brain, which can cause symptoms of anxiety and fatigue. Some people think that sleep apnea occurs in people who are overweight. This is definitely a trend; however, plenty of people of all sizes struggle with sleep apnea. And many people who receive corrective therapy for sleep apnea report that their fatigue, anxiety, and depression improve greatly. Healthy sleeping has the added benefit of giving them more energy to address their anxiety and make better food choices to better regulate their glucose. Many people don't want to explore sleep apnea because they don't like the treatment: using a continuous positive airway pressure (CPAP) device. A CPAP device uses a mask that fits over the nose and/or mouth, and gently blows air into the airway to help keep people breathing consistently throughout the night.

Rather than avoiding the treatment, if you think you may have sleep apnea, try the following experiments before you reject the treatment.

Experiments to Address Snoring

- Try sleeping with nasal strips for 10 to 14 days.

- Ask your primary care physician for a referral to a sleep clinic for a sleep assessment.

Did you try one of the above? What did you learn? Did it help?

Why Can't I Get Out of Bed?

When people complain about not being able to get out of bed in the morning, we ask them why they *want* to get out of bed. The answer is often a long list of shoulds and have-to's ("I have to go to work, I have to take care of the kids, I have to do this, I have to do that…"). But what in their day or week or month do they do because they *want* to? Because it excites them? Quite often, the same people who have a hard time getting out of bed are the ones who rarely do things they enjoy. A lot of people have the tendency to downplay their passions. When talking about their passions, people may sheepishly admit that they're a huge fan of the *Lord of the Rings* trilogy or share other confessions about innocuous interests and guilty pleasures. We really don't care if you spent three years researching everything about a movie or anything else that you have found interesting enough to learn deeply about. Yet there's a deep sense of shame if we think that our passions somehow don't measure up to a sense of societal worthiness. On some level, these simple passions are shunned in our society. So the question is, *Why get out of bed?*

Experiments in Putting Things You Enjoy Back into Your Life

- Make a list of past hobbies and pleasures that you engaged in as a kid or young adult, and write out the first two steps that it would take to engage in them again.

- Set aside time in your calendar, even if it's just ten minutes, for you to focus on something you enjoy, something to look forward to.

- Are there friends or family members who enjoy the same activities you do? Can you find ways to do them together?

- Connect to groups that have activities, such as the YMCA, universities or colleges, and Meetups (http://www.meetup.com).

What actions are you going to take to add your passions back into your life?

Feel Safe When Sleeping

Many people with anxiety and sleep challenges have histories of trauma. If they were abused, even if they're safe now, they may still have a hard time feeling safe while they sleep. The problem is, when we sleep, we can be at any time and any place. We can revisit the sensations of the past as if it were today. Giving the body an "anchor" to today—something that we can be aware of in the background while we sleep—can be very helpful. The anchor needs to be something that isn't part of the past. While we sleep, our subconscious monitors the present moment as well as revisits the past. Kristen has found in her clinical practice that when people with a history of trauma take concrete actions to create a sense of safety by identifying an anchor that works for them, their quality of sleep can be greatly improved.

Here are some anchors that people have used:

- A cardboard refrigerator box, sealed with duct tape and having only one entrance, filled with blankets and pillows and decorated on the inside, became the safe space to sleep.

- Installing a lock on the bedroom door, with an extra key for a partner who might enter later in the night, ensured that no one without permission could enter the bedroom.

- Tying a string around the bedroom doorknob and connecting it to a bedside lamp so it would crash down if the door were opened at night ensured that a sound would wake the sleeper and scare off any intruders.

- Wrapping hands with ACE bandages while sleeping has served as a reminder that the sleeper is safe from past injuries.

It's not what you *think* is safe; it's what will make you *feel* safe. If you can sleep feeling really safe for a while, sleeping through the night will become more of a habit. Can you think of some things to try to increase your feeling of safety while you sleep?

Now that you've learned more about the importance of good sleep and some ways to improve the quality and quantity of sleep, let's see how Luca implements them in her busy life.

Luca Prepares to Meet with Clients the Next Day

After Luca gets the kids to bed, she's tempted to have a glass of wine to relax. But after talking with her sister, she wonders if that is part of what's causing her to wake up at 3:00 a.m. with anxiety and racing thoughts. She skips the wine and focuses on tomorrow. She decides that she's going to do everything she can to set herself up for success and starts to think it through.

Her alarm will go off at 6:00 a.m., so she wants to be asleep by 10:00 p.m. to get eight hours of sleep, which she knows will help her. She decides that she will get ready for bed at 9:30 p.m. to give herself some time to read a book that has encouraging stories before she falls asleep. Her sister suggested that she eat protein before going to bed. After looking around her kitchen, she decides that the easiest choice is to eat a scoop of peanut butter. She also plans to put juice and nuts by her bed in case she wakes up in the middle of the night. And if she sleeps through the night, Luca plans to drink the juice before getting out of bed in the morning to help orient her brain.

Next, she rummages around the kitchen for an idea for breakfast. She finds a protein shake that she got for her son a couple of weeks ago. That will be her breakfast. Thinking through her day, she realizes that if she drinks the shake at 6:30 a.m., with the excitement of the meeting, she'll also need to be sure to have a snack before 10:00 a.m. to control the amount of adrenaline in her system. There's a deli near work, and Luca decides to get a turkey sandwich that she will eat around 9:30 a.m. Luca knows that she'll feel more confident if she can review the material before the meeting, so she texts a trusted coworker, James, to see if they can meet at 9:00 a.m. to review the project. James quickly responds that he's available.

Luca decides to write all of this out in a list, so she won't worry about forgetting her plan.

☐ Protein before bed

☐ Juice and nuts on bed stand

☐ 6:00: Wake up and drink ¼ cup of juice

☐ 6:30: Protein shake and wake the kids

☐ 7:30: Get kids to school

☐ 7:45: Leave for work

☐ 8:00: Buy turkey sandwich at deli and look at email

☐ 9:00: Meet with James

☐ 9:30: Eat ½ sandwich

☐ 10:00: Meeting with boss and clients

☐ After meeting: call sister

The next morning, Luca wakes up with her alarm. She's a little startled that she did not wake up in the middle of the night. She definitely feels awake and decides not to have the juice; she's actually hungry and is relieved that she knows the protein shake is waiting for her and that she doesn't have to think about what to feed herself. Organizing the kids for school goes a little easier than normal; Luca wonders if it's because she fed herself first.

When she gets to work, she's already thinking about talking with James and the client meeting. Because of this internal conversation, she walks right past the deli. It's not until she's at her office door that she remembers she wanted to buy a turkey sandwich on her way in. In this moment, she feels good. Part of her says, "Skip it, you're fine; go clear your email." She has heard that voice *before, and she knows that she can be fine now and in a couple of hours be on the verge of a panic attack. She walks back to buy the sandwich. In her office, Luca gets out her list and starts checking things off. The conversation with James goes well. He's encouraging. When he asks about her plan, she shares that she is going to fuel her brain before the meeting to see if that makes it easier to manage her anxiety. When they wrap up, she eats half of her sandwich and walks to the conference room.*

She's fifteen minutes early and takes a moment to focus on what's happening right now: the window opens to a beautiful sky, and the room is quiet. She finds a small moment in which she can relax into her body. Luca assumes that her boss will bring in the client; however, as she is sitting there gathering her thoughts, the client walks in and reintroduces herself. They chat a little about the weather. Luca notices that although her anxiety went up a little when her client came in, she can tell that the client is relaxed. Maybe she's not really in trouble. Her boss walks in, and there is more chitchat. Then, she turns to Luca and says, "Why don't you update us on the project." Luca looks at her notes for a moment and freezes. But she can hear her boss's voice from last night, "Just present what you shared last week. It's just an update."

Luca takes a breath and starts. There's a light back-and-forth. Luca actually notices that she smiles during the presentation. The client has some questions. Luca doesn't have answers for two of the questions and suggests that she can email the client later in the week. The client is fine with this! After about thirty minutes, her boss thanks her for the review and dismisses her while the two of them continue on other projects. Luca walks out of the room thinking, That went fine, maybe even better than fine. *As soon as she is in the stairwell of the office building, Luca calls her sister. "I did it! I was nervous but not anxious. The meeting went well. I think paying attention to how I fuel my body and my brain really helped."*

CHAPTER SUMMARY

Understanding what disrupts your sleep and how to improve your sleep is essential to getting a good night's rest and having a stable power supply. Two sleep worksheets are available in the appendix and at http://www.newharbinger.com/46233.

In the next chapter, we'll explain how movement also supports your power supply.

## CHAPTER 8

Moving Your Body for More Energy and Mental Clarity

Exercise is another aspect of your behavior and lifestyle that can help you make real progress with anxiety, worry, and fatigue. If you don't exercise but want to start, this chapter will have some suggestions to help you get started. If you don't exercise and don't want to exercise, please don't skip this chapter. There are times not to start an exercise program, but there's a huge benefit to starting small and slow. Finally, if you're already exercising, we'll encourage you to continue and suggest new ways to integrate movement into your life.

In this chapter we're going to talk about moving your body for a very specific outcome: to have more energy and mental clarity. We're going to say this again: the goal of this chapter is for you to have tools for movement that you trust to consistently increase your *energy and mental clarity*. This is very different from goals around losing weight or preventing a negative outcome, like diabetes or cardiovascular disease. These benefits may be attained over time with our system, but what we have seen over and over is that when people aren't focused on using movement to feel better, they don't sustain the activity, and they're prone to injury. But when movement is used to improve our daily lives, the practice can be sustained, built on, and enjoyed. Movement provides a very clear path for addressing the physiological underpinnings of anxiety and fatigue (Ratey and Hagerman 2008). We provide experiments that will help you feel this effect in as little as 30 seconds, with longer-lasting resilience coming from experiments lasting for 30 days.

There are three key takeaways of this chapter:

1. **Three elements for an achievable movement plan for everyone**. We provide experiments for each element that are focused on increasing movement for more energy and mental clarity.

2. **Barriers for movement.** There are many unrecognized reasons for why people choose not to move their bodies, outside of daily activities. It's very important to address these reasons when establishing a new movement plan.

3. **Minimal metrics for movement.** Physical independence is so important to our self-identity. Understanding what your current minimal metrics are is one way to ensure continued freedom and hope.

MOVEMENT VERSUS "EXERCISE"

There are a lot of words used to describe intentionally moving your body: movement, physical activity, exercise, play, rehab or physical therapy, conditioning, toning, strengthening, coordination, and balance, to name a few. All of these tend to be emotionally loaded in some way and are quite often focused around gaining something that we don't have or have lost. The word "exercise," in particular, is rarely equated with improving energy and mental clarity. For many people, exercise is more often equated with weight loss. Because of this, as we move forward, we use the word "movement" since it's the broadest term—meaning anything that uses skeletal muscles and the skeletal structure to intentionally move your body. In the context of movement, depending on who you are, you might have an exercise program, or you might need a rehab program. You might just define this as your "waypower" program or as play.

First, we'd like you to take a moment to think about what word or words resonate with you. What is your word that makes the activity of moving your body feel accessible? It's really important that you define this for yourself in a way that makes it meaningful to your situation, to specifically support increased energy and mental clarity, and to increase the freedom you feel in your body and in your life. *Everyone* can work toward this. We're asking you to think about the words you use because we're explicitly asking you to change your intention around movement so that you're focused on increasing energy and mental clarity instead of all the other reasons that might bubble up in your mind. We don't really care which word or words work for you; we just want you to capture this intention. Check off any of the below words you're comfortable using that you can associate with feeling more resilient in your life. Add to this list if you want to.

☐ Conditioning: developing broader abilities to move your body

☐ Coordination: practicing patterns of movement that require balance, core muscle strength, and opposite sides of the body

☐ Embodiment: trusting the impulse of your body to respond in the moment

☐ Exercise: repetitive and intentional movement

☐ Flexibility: moving joints and muscles to maintain range of motion and resilience

☐ Movement: intentional movement of your body to have more energy and mental clarity

☐ Play: moving your body for enjoyment

☐ Practice: a movement performed regularly to discover what is possible in that moment

☐ Rehab: recovering or developing functionality of a specific area of the body

☐ Strengthening/bodybuilding: moving muscle sets to increase muscle strength

☐ _____

☐ _____

☐ _____

Now that we have a better sense of the different kinds of movement that you want to focus on, let's look at the three elements of our movement plan.

THREE ELEMENTS OF A MOVEMENT PLAN

Whether they know it or not, everyone alive has a movement plan. We need to move our bodies to feed ourselves, to go to work or school, to engage with family and friends, to travel, and to enjoy being alive. The movement plan we present here supports people who want to figure out how to expand on what they're already doing by integrating more movement throughout their day. We provide tools to increase not only the dexterity of your body but also the neuroplasticity of your brain so that you can have more energy and mental clarity and less worry, anxiety, and stress.

The three elements of this movement plan are:

1. 30-second Power-Ups.

2. Walking for an hour.

3. Finding something that you love.

As we explain each element of the movement plan in detail, we offer experiments for you to try. But first, how do you recognize that you have more energy and mental clarity? What does this mean to *you*? It's important to think about this up front because if we do have more energy and mental clarity, we might use it only to fulfill our to-do lists. Ironically, sometimes being fatigued may actually help you be less anxious because it lowers the expectation of what *can* be done.

Having more energy and mental clarity gives us the capacity to have our minds run the show, rather than our reactive brains. This means that we have better capacity to be curious about our lives, to be self-compassionate for being human, to see the factors that are influencing our lives, and, importantly, to make choices to increase our own well-being and resilience. How this shows up for each individual is different. Some common observations include sustained energy levels throughout the day, increased ability to keep commitments, ability to pay better attention, less drive to binge or engage in other negative behaviors, and increased ability to engage in self-care and personal interests.

For Kristen, on the days that she walks 10 to 15 minutes in the morning, she is able to get her clinical notes done while the patient is in the room or in the time before her next patient. When she doesn't, she spends 45 to 60 minutes charting at the end of the day. It took a month of morning walks for Kristen to see the correlation. Once she made that connection, she realized that the benefit of taking some time out every morning for a little movement was immediate. Natasha notices a different pattern. When she makes time to move her body in the morning, she finds she has enough energy after work to enjoy making dinner, instead of throwing something in the microwave or toaster oven and plopping down in front of the TV.

Naming why you want to change, or what you'll do with more energy and less anxiety, can be a powerful motivator for investing time and energy in an activity. Think about how having energy and mental clarity and increased physical ability to engage in your life might increase your resilience.

Set Yourself Up for Being Inconsistently Consistent

We're so tired of the discussion about how much exercise we need to get. Studies show that we "need" 150 minutes of exercise per week to get the maximum health benefits. The problem with this metric is that it doesn't provide a tangible place to start from. And if you're out of shape, have a health condition that makes it seem impossible to meet that mark, or are just too tired to get started, a goal like this can make it hard to even try.

It's also not a great metric in and of itself for people who are hitting that 150-minute mark per week. When people engage in the same type of exercise (jogging, walking, jumping rope, and so forth) week after week and year after year, it becomes less effective over time because they don't stay as engaged in the activity as they once did—it takes less brain effort and less physical effort to get it done. Engaging in the same exercise, without challenging both body and mind, reduces the positive impact of movement on energy, mental clarity, and resilience.

When we're asked how much movement someone should do, we use these guidelines to help people identify a doable starting place for themselves:

1. **Consistently do something most days of the week.** If we want to work out four days a week, we likely have to schedule it for six days a week or we'll end up doing it only twice. In our busy lives, it seems almost inevitable that something unplanned will come up about twice a week that interferes with our schedules. Recognizing this means that we can plan for it!

2. **Do the amount of movement that does not cause pain or fatigue.** Remember: we're looking for more energy and mental clarity in the present moment; the rest will come with time! It's okay to be a little tired after moving your body, but if you're significantly fatigued or in pain, then the "dose" is too high.

Instead of starting out by focusing on how far you walked or how many reps you did, we encourage you to start by simply creating a time to move your body and then showing up for it. The very beginning may not always be enjoyable because your brain may come up with all sorts of explanations for why you shouldn't or don't have time to move your body. For example, focus on just showing up for movement for 30 days, even if it takes 45 to 60 days to hit that mark. This is what we call being inconsistently consistent, which means that you keep showing up even if it's not perfect or if you miss a day. Remember that your focus during this time is to use movement to improve energy, mental clarity, resilience, and freedom to engage with the world in a more meaningful way.

It helps to find ways to mark how many times you show up for movement. People who do this are often more likely to keep up the habit. One technique is to use an "I did it" vase or a bowl. Each time you find a way to intentionally move your body, put a rock, a penny, a piece of beach glass, or some other small object in the container. As you do this over time, you'll see the volume of what you have done.

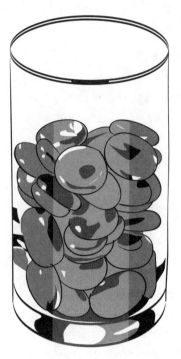

WHAT IS THE RIGHT "DOSE" OF MOVEMENT FOR YOU RIGHT NOW?

- Generally, an appropriate amount of movement may result in feeling slightly physically tired but otherwise fine; ideally, you'll feel mentally relaxed after activity. The next day you might be a little tight, but not physically or mentally tired.

- Too much movement results in feeling sore and both physically and mentally tired following the movement, and possibly for the next couple of days.

- If you can't find an exercise level that is comfortable, seek the assistance of a doctor, physical therapist, or physical fitness trainer.

Let's see how simple it is to start.

Element 1: 30-Second Power-Ups, Every Day, Throughout the Day

One of Kristen's favorite activities as a public speaker is to do an experiment with the audience to see if they can experience an improvement in their energy and mental clarity in thirty seconds. Most of the room reports that they get at least a 10 percent bump in their power supply after doing the activity.

Here's the experiment she asks them to do: Rate your current power supply, and then stand up and choose one of the following four movements that you're most comfortable doing, for a count of four: (1) chair squats, (2) marching in place, (3) wall push-ups, or (4) clapping over your head. We call these activities "Power-Ups" because they increase your physical and mental energy and are easy to do anywhere.

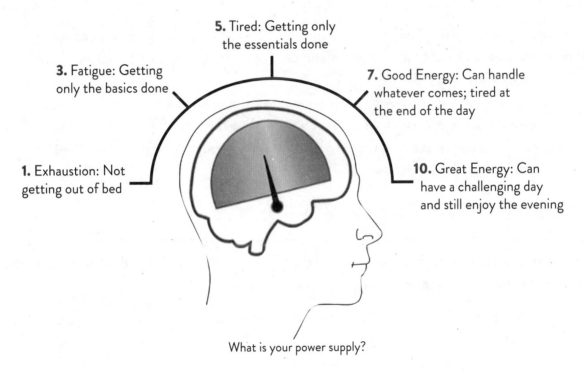

5. Tired: Getting only the essentials done

3. Fatigue: Getting only the basics done

7. Good Energy: Can handle whatever comes; tired at the end of the day

1. Exhaustion: Not getting out of bed

10. Great Energy: Can have a challenging day and still enjoy the evening

What is your power supply?

WHAT IS A POWER-UP?

A Power-Up is a quick activity that

- Is easy to do

- Takes as little as 30 seconds, and no more than five minutes or so

- Can be done in all sorts of places without changing your clothes

- Doesn't increase pain or fatigue

- Intentionally and repetitively uses your muscles

- Probably won't cause you to break a sweat

Do your chosen activity for a count of 1…2…3…4, and then sit down and rerate your power supply. Was there a change? Most people are surprised to realize that, if they started the activity at a 6 (out of 10), they now feel like they're at a 7 or 8.

Starting this small is an accessible way for you to get a little taste of the tangible benefits of moving even if you struggle with willingness. Think about it this way: if you could get a 10 percent raise in salary at a cost of just 10 minutes a day, would it be worth it? Most people say, "Yes!"

Are you ready to experiment with Power-Ups?

THE 30-SECOND POWER-UP EXPERIMENT

Are you willing to try something for just 30 seconds? Until people are able to feel the effect in their own bodies, some may dismiss this as "not enough to be worth doing." You don't have to do the activities we list, but getting what they represent is important.

1. Check in and rate your power supply at this moment. _____

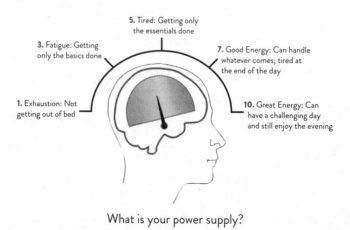

5. Tired: Getting only the essentials done

3. Fatigue: Getting only the basics done

7. Good Energy: Can handle whatever comes; tired at the end of the day

1. Exhaustion: Not getting out of bed

10. Great Energy: Can have a challenging day and still enjoy the evening

What is your power supply?

2. Now stand up. Choose one of the Power-Up movements that you will do for a count of four (1...2...3...4).

    ◆ **Chair squats.** Have a chair behind you and sit down as though you are going to take a seat. Just as you touch the chair, stand back up.

    ◆ **March in place.** March with your knees coming up as high as it's comfortable.

    ◆ **Wall push-ups.** Place your hands on a wall with your feet about arm's-length away from the wall; bend your arms until your nose is near the wall or you think you're close enough; push back out to an extended arm position.

    ◆ **Overhead hand clap.** Raise both arms in the air and bring your hands together comfortably over your head. Clap your hands together if that sounds like fun.

    Remember: do one of these, just four times.

3. Sit back down and rerate your power supply. _____

If you were initially at 6 (out of 10), you might now be at 7...in less than thirty seconds! What could you do with consistently 10 percent more energy?

There are multiple benefits to Power-Ups. Studies show that sitting continuously for extended periods of time (more than seven hours per day) shortens your life by creating conditions for anxiety, depression, cardiovascular disease, and diabetes (Chau et al. 2013; Stanczykiewicz et al. 2019). However, having small moments of movement can positively impact people's lives and reduce these risks. A few minutes of movement each hour have been shown to improve both physical well-being and cognitive functioning (Dregan and Gulliford 2013). Again, most people experience an improvement in their energy level by at least 10 percent. And some people realize the reason they often get up to get coffee or something sweet isn't actually that they need those things, but that they need some movement, and walking to get them is effectively a Power-Up.

Get more ideas for Power-Ups from sites like YouTube, by searching for:

- Balance exercises
- Coordination exercises
- Sprinting in place
- Core exercises, such as the dead bug
- Overhead arm clap
- Office exercises, desk exercises, chair yoga.

We also have Power-Up examples at http://www.kristenallott.com/blog.

Remember: figure out what gives you an immediate energy boost, start at your comfort level, and have fun with it!

What's more, the cumulative impact of moving our bodies raises our self-esteem and resilience. The difference of doing purposeful movement to improve our well-being, even as small as a Power-Up, can create significant positive impacts on quality of life over time. Brain-derived neurotrophic factor has been shown to be low in people with conditions like anxiety and depression (Suliman, Hemmings, and Seedat 2013). Moving skeletal muscles releases brain-derived neurotrophic factor (brain fertilizer), which helps with learning, energy, and mental clarity (Smits et al. 2016).

What different Power-Ups do for you.

- *Chair squats* build the muscle strength required to do a controlled sit and a controlled rise out of a chair. When people start by doing a count of 4, building to a count of 10, sitting and standing up from chairs becomes easier over time.

- *Wall push-ups* build upper-body strength, which is often ignored. The nice thing about wall push-ups is that you can do them against any wall, a closed and locked door, or a door frame. Wall push-ups eliminate the barrier of getting down on the floor and reduce the portion of body weight that you're moving. Over time, as you get stronger, you can move to a more horizontal position by using a chair or couch that is up against a wall.

- *Marching in place* briefly increases your heart rate and breathing, circulating nutrients throughout your body and brain. Bringing your knees as high up as comfortable builds your skills, including balance for walking. It's also a great way to activate your body after sitting. An easy way to build the amount of time you engage in this Power-Up is to put on a favorite song and march to it. Another variation is walking up and down stairs.

- *Clapping your hands over your head,* in a sitting or standing position, activates the muscles holding your head up, increases blood flow, strengthens your upper body, and ultimately makes sitting more comfortable.

How to build a Power-Up program. It's important to start with what you're most comfortable with and then add Power-Ups that help you improve on specific skills. Things that happen together wire together in the brain. So, if you want to get better at comfortably standing and sitting, chair squats are a good place to start. If your lower body is injured right now, you can still move your upper body by starting with clapping overhead or wall push-ups. Remember, you're doing this to improve energy and mental clarity first. Until you have improved your power supply, it's very hard to address patterns of pain and restriction. We want you to start well beneath these thresholds and with activities that are accessible to your body now.

Find moments throughout the day that you can insert a Power-Up. Be playful. Where can you place these Power-Ups to improve your day? Before a meeting? After a meeting? Before picking up the kids from school? Before or after you get in or out of a car? In the bathroom? When you get off the couch from watching TV?

As you begin working Power-Ups into your day-to-day life, experiment with the number of times you can comfortably do each movement. What happens if you do six instead of four? What happens if you do 10? What happens if you do your Power-Ups four or five times in the same day?

Once you get into the routine of adding Power-Ups throughout the day, add variety in the type of Power-Ups you do. List 10 places where you could do a Power-Up.

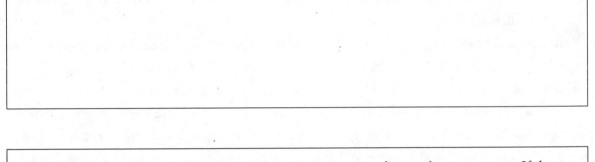

When to seek help. Pain and fatigue are two primary reasons for avoiding movement. If this is true for you, you may need to start by addressing these issues with your primary care provider. If you're in pain, talk with your provider about how you can safely work toward improving your health amid the pain. This may include working with a physical therapist on specific movements; a physical therapist can help build specific Power-Ups for your individual needs. By assembling a team, you can reduce your anxiety about not being resilient in the world.

To conclude element 1, if you haven't exercised for a while, it might take weeks, months, or a year to build these skills. That's okay! Give yourself permission to add this small bit of movement into your day, at whatever level you can, and you'll see improvement over time. We list Power-Ups as the first element of the movement plan because if you can't do Power-Ups, walking for an hour will likely be hard. If you're already moving your body regularly, these are a great way to increase your overall movement and energy level throughout the day.

Element 2: Build a Base of Walking

Our ancestors did a lot of walking. Walking is one of the basic movements that supports physical and mental health, and it improves the functionality of the brain through many different mechanisms: it releases brain-derived neurotrophic factor, increases blood flow, decreases cortisol, decreases inflammation, and improves glucose regulation, among others (Kandola et al. 2018). By building a base of walking, you'll improve the strength of your lower body, your core, and your back muscles, all of which help release muscle tension and improve digestion. Walking also strengthens the heart and improves the quality of sleep. Importantly, walking seems to provide a way to process what is happening in our lives because it uses both the right and left hemispheres of the brain. Walking reduces worry and anxiety by improving your sense of independence and security and increasing your ability to engage in life in the manner that you want. Building a base of walking is a key activity to maintain throughout all stages of life.

Kristen and Natasha share the goal of being able to comfortably walk three miles in under an hour. We have both had the experience where we were working out three to five times per week—Natasha doing an at-home fitness exercise routine and Kristen doing Aikido, a defensive martial art—but when we had to walk a distance, we were sore. Why was that? Well, walking uses a particular set of muscles, and we were missing them in our weekly routines. This is one of the reasons that we need to have variety in what we do so that we are using most of our muscles and as many systems in the brain as possible.

Benefits of Adding 10 Minutes of Walking to an Existing Movement Program

- If you work out in the evening, walking for 10 minutes in the morning can increase your energy and mental clarity and reduce anxiety throughout the day.

- Walking for 10 minutes midday can reduce afternoon fatigue and situational anxiety.

- Walking can also provide a time out during stressful situations, which can help reduce anxiety.

- Walking provides a sense of control by making a choice of where to walk.

- Walking provides new input to the brain, which sometimes leads to a new perspective on a situation.

- Walking outside can decrease stress hormones.

Generally, we recommend that you start with 10 minutes of walking per day and a personal commitment to a number of days within a set period of time. For example, if your goal is to walk for 10 minutes a day for 30 days, give yourself 45 days to accomplish this. Here's why: our brains resist doing new things that we don't have a lot of experience with or that have been negative in the past. If you've been moving your body just to get things done, you likely don't know what the reward is, so your brain is going to urge you *not* to do it: *You have other things to do, You have a program to watch,* or whatever your inner dialogue comes up with. This is the value of doing a movement experiment: You can say to the resistance, *We are only doing 10 minutes a day most days. If we feel no different after we meet our goal, then we can stop.*

Also, it's a simple truth that things will come up in your life and you'll miss some days of walking. Remember, if your goal is to walk five times a week, you'll likely need to schedule it seven times. Missing those two extra times isn't failure! It's working movement into your life in a realistic way by enabling you to hit your target through the practice of being inconsistently consistent. We suggest the target of practicing walking for 30 days within a 45-day period, because it will take about 30 days to create a new movement habit and to discover the dose and pattern that work for you. For some people, 10 minutes might be too long; they'll get sore and too tired, and maybe starting with three minutes of walking a day is a better entry place. Others who start with 10 minutes find that they enjoy it, that it feels good, and that they want to go for longer time periods sooner. The nice thing about 10 minutes a day, for people building their conditioning, is that usually they find after 30 days that they can walk further within the 10 minutes. This adds to their confidence.

HOW TO TOLERATE WALKING

Generally, our brains are conditioned to think we need to always be doing something. Having a plan for what we can do to occupy our brains while walking is important. Using more than one option is also important to prevent boredom. Here are some ideas:

- Listen to music, a podcast, or audiobook.

- Call a friend or family member.

- Walk with a neighbor, friend, or pet.

- Create a mindfulness practice while walking. For example, use your senses to name what you see, hear, and feel. This helps your brain practice being in the present moment. Here are some questions to ask yourself while you walk:

    - What colors do I see? Track one color each day: red, blue, yellow, green, white, and so on. You may be surprised by how much a specific color is around in different seasons.

    - Can I hear what's happening around me, such as birdsongs? Try to listen for the more subtle noises that you may often filter out or ignore.

    - Does the temperature of the air seem to change as I walk? For instance, it might be cooler under a tree.

- Use the walk to accomplish a goal, such as walking to the store, taking photographs, or visiting a friend. One woman decided to take a picture of a tree in the small park that she would walk around near her work. Each day she went for her 15-minute walk and took a picture. From day to day, it was hard to see the changes, but over the course of a year, she had captured all the fall colors and the hibernation of the winter, and she discovered that the buds of spring started in the gloom of February in Seattle. By the time she was in the midst of the vibrancy of spring, she recognized her own vibrancy returning. She then put her 98 photos together into a slide deck to show the changes. What was nice about taking the photos is that she knew they represented 98 walking sessions. And, like the tree, at first it was hard to notice the change, but as the movement accumulated, she could tell she had less anxiety, less fatigue, and more confidence.

What can you do when you go out for a walk? How do you plan to monitor for the cumulative effect? Remember that it's helpful to have more than one choice.

EXPERIMENTS WITH WALKING

For the walking experiment, we're going to take you through a few questions to help you shape your own experiment because everyone is different. For this experiment, your goal is to have more energy and mental clarity and less anxiety and worry; other benefits will come along with time, but this is a good starting point.

1. Rate your power supply: _____ .   Rate your anxiety range during the week: _____

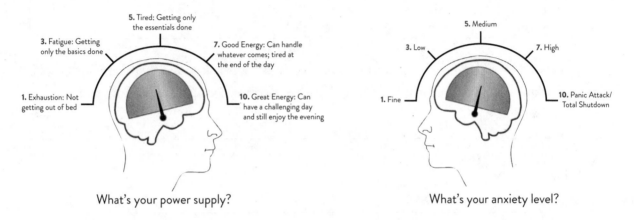

What's your power supply?   What's your anxiety level?

2. How long or far can you comfortably walk right now, without causing discomfort in any way?

Can you already walk for 10 minutes? If not, you might set a distance goal: to a mailbox, the corner, a loop around the house, or whatever other mark feels right.

3. What time, or times, will you add this activity into your day? Give yourself permission for it to end up being inconsistently consistent.

4. How many times are you willing to commit to the experiment? Our recommendation is to hit 30 days within a 45-day period. However, that might not be realistic in your life. Please make a realistic goal for yourself. You don't have to wait for a "free" 45-day period! Just extend the 45 days to however long you need in order to hit the mark of walking 30 separate times.

```
[                                                                    ]
```

5. How will you monitor the number of times you walk? We have found that, for many people, marking it on a calendar isn't effective. Consider creating a visually tangible system, such as an "I did it" vase.

```
[                                                                    ]
```

6. What will you do when you go out for a walk to keep yourself interested in the activity?

```
[                                                                    ]
```

You're ready to begin! As you're doing the experiment, here are some things to think about. Our brains are more likely to want to repeat doing something if we talk about it or share it. Some people like to share that they're doing a walking experiment and what they're noticing with family members, friends, or a therapist. Other people are more private about their experiments, which is fine too! If you're not sharing with people in your life, at the end of the day be sure to share with yourself through journaling or by naming to yourself what you remember about the walk. This doesn't have to be done every time, but reflecting on your walking practice will reinforce your adoption of it.

How are you going to reinforce the activity of walking?

```


```

7. Now that you're into the experiment… Have you gone for a walk 10 to 20 times yet? Some people notice differences in how they feel right away, and others take longer to feel the effects. Both are okay! The important thing is to keep checking in with yourself throughout the experiment. And remember not to make decisions about the utility of the experiment until the end because you don't know if how you feel will change over time.

   Have you noticed changes in how you feel in your body and mind since you began the experiment? Have you noticed if you can walk more comfortably or farther within the same time frame? Did you stay with your original time frame, or were there times you walked for longer or shorter? Has tracking the number of times you've walked given you a sense of accomplishment?

```


```

8. You did it—you completed 30 days of walking! Congratulations! What happened over the course of the experiment? Let's check back in with the questions you answered at the beginning.

1. Rate your power supply: _____   Rate your anxiety range during the week: _____

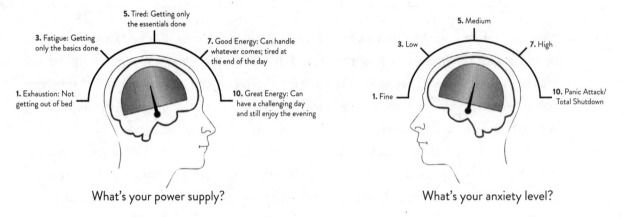

What's your power supply?   What's your anxiety level?

2. If you were feeling discomfort while walking at first: How long or far can you comfortably walk right now without causing discomfort in any way? Has this changed since the beginning of the experiment?

3. What else have you noticed that has changed since you started walking more regularly? Common things are that Power-Ups are easier to do, your anxiety is lower, your sleep is better, and your self-confidence may have improved. Remember that these are just some of the things that people notice—it's okay if what you experience is different.

4. Do you plan to continue a practice of walking? _____

Now that you've completed this experiment in walking, what's your next experiment? Hopefully walking in an inconsistently consistent way has increased your energy and mental clarity and reduced your anxiety and worry. It's important to create a plan or further experiments to continue to have these benefits. One option is to repeat the same walking experiment or to change the duration, distance, or frequency that you walk. Regardless of whatever else you decide to do, continuing to build your walking skill will always be important because of the freedom, independence, and confidence that comes from it. Maybe a mile or 20 minutes is good enough. Maybe you want to explore historic sites around the world, so you may want to build up to three or even six miles. Kristen and her husband try to walk for two hours every Sunday. They mostly just wander around different parts of their hometown.

What place will walking have in your life?

Element 3: Building the Life You Want to Live

Earlier in this workbook, we asked you what you want to do when you have more energy and mental clarity, your anxiety is more under control, and you have a better power supply to engage in your life. If you felt more hope in your life, what would you do? Travel, garden, go back to school, change to a more supportive job environment, redecorate your house? What are your long-term goals, and what level of physical fitness will you need? Building and maintaining physical fitness will determine how many adventures you get to go on and how well you weather health crises. As we move into each decade of life, we need to put more effort into maintaining our physical and psychological well-being. We're more successful at this if we set up our lifestyles to include movement activities that we enjoy doing to ensure we reap the benefits.

ADDING DIVERSITY TO YOUR MOVEMENT ACTIVITIES

Once people have built a base of walking and hopefully are still practicing the Power-Ups, we generally encourage them to look for another form of movement unique to them that they find to be fun, interesting, or socially supportive. We suggest that people look into the YMCA or local gym; you might also consider looking at what's available locally through http://www.meetup.com, as there are often groups for walking, cycling, dance, mini golf, or tai chi (among others!). If you're not sure what you would really enjoy doing, try several activities, such as beginners' groups, to find a good fit. Another approach is to commit to trying a new activity at least three times before rejecting it: the first time you go, your brain will say, "That was awful!" because the unfamiliarity might feel uncomfortable. The second time, you'll have more familiarity, but not enough to notice what you enjoy or what might be appealing to you. The third time, you can start paying more attention to what might keep you engaged in the activity for a three- to six-month trial.

We're always surprised at the different activities people decide to stick with. One man decided on long-distance biking purely by accident; he was on a bike, left his neighborhood, and stopped when he reached the next city 35 miles later. One woman in her seventies took up kung fu at a local dojo, and the younger people there enjoyed having a grandma (who could beat them up). Another woman started walking 10Ks as part of her vacation planning and in the process made friends throughout the country and now around the world.

Experiments to Help You Find Things You Love to Do

1. **Make a list of at least 20 things** available near the different locations where you spend time, on a blank piece of paper. Notice, the activity isn't "list things that you're interested in doing." This is an opportunity to consider new things. We often have to do the thing before we know if we want to continue to do it. It might take up to a week to find twenty activities, and that's okay. Take some time to ponder it; be creative! You might include using the StairMaster at a local gym, joining a weightlifting class, taking swim classes, playing racquetball, attending Meetup walking or jogging groups, trying

> **Multiple Benefits from a Single Activity**
>
> Part of what kept Kristen in Aikido, a defensive martial art, is that in addition to providing a workout and interesting personal learning curve, it was also a friendship group, it taught mindfulness, and it counted as her spiritual practice. On different days, different benefits were emphasized, which kept her engaged.

YouTube workout programs, participating in university or parks and recreational programs, or joining an adult recreational league (softball, soccer). Don't worry about prioritizing your list yet—we'll get to that in the next step.

- Can you work it into your schedule?

- Is it available every day, on specific days, or in certain seasons (for example, snow skiing)?

- Is it something you will do on your own or would prefer to do it with a friend? We will often commit to other people before we commit to ourselves, so finding someone to do a new activity with might help you sustain the commitment.

- Are there multiple benefits to participating in a specific activity?

- How does cost motivate you or restrict you from participating in the activity? Knowing the cost of starting a new activity is important. Some people find that investing in an activity (for example, buying a 10-class yoga pass) can motivate them to follow through.

- Are there simple solutions to perceived barriers? For example, Natasha, who works from home, realized that if she started the day wearing walking shoes, she was much more likely to actually hop on the elliptical trainer while she was on the phone or listening to a podcast than if she stayed in her slippers.

2. **Add your list to the activities chart** (below, in the appendix, and at http://www.newharbin ger.com/46233). This will help you differentiate the activities on your list. We had you start on a blank piece of paper because we didn't want you to do a lot of analysis as you were making your list. This helps you be more creative in the initial phase.

Activities Chart	Convenience (location)	Convenience (timing)	Available every day	Available some days	Available in specific seasons	Would do alone	Would do only with a friend	Multiple benefits	Needs special gear	Other	Rank
1.											
2.											
3.											
4.											
5.											
6.											
7.											
8.											
9.											
10.											
11.											
12.											
13.											
14.											
15.											
16.											
17.											
18.											
19.											
20.											

3. **Based on the chart, what are the top three to five activities you're willing to try?** If you don't feel you have enough information to choose, try a couple of the activities. Notice if you feel that it's physically safe and if the teacher, if there is one, can accommodate your skill level or physical abilities. Talk with the instructor about your goals and their expectations; talk with others engaging in the activity to get their points of view. Are you willing to try the activity three times? You may decide to stay with the first activity, or you may decide to try a few different things before committing—both paths are fine.

4. **Now you're ready to start the experiment of finding new things to love! Let's make a plan.**

   ☐ Place it in your schedule: add it to your work and/or family calendar.

   ☐ Assemble workout clothes or equipment you might need in a bag.

   ☐ Make a commitment (to yourself or someone else) for how many times you're going to engage in the activity before you decide that it's not for you; three is the bare minimum.

   ☐ List the conditions under which you'll stop before meeting this commitment, for example, if you feel unsafe (physically or emotionally), you're in increased pain, or you're overly fatigued the next day.

   ☐ Identify the reward you get for completing the experiment. Some people use stickers, a chocolate truffle, new workout clothes, or something special to add to their "I did it" vase. It's nice to pat yourself on the back for doing something you might be reluctant to try.

5. **You did it!** What are the things you learned by completing this experiment? What did you enjoy? Not enjoy? Did it help your energy and mental clarity and decrease your anxiety? What's your next movement experiment going to be?

Hopefully you've been able to start experimenting with these new tools and are feeling the benefits in both your body and brain. Movement is a lifelong practice. With Power-Ups, walking, and seeking diversity in your movement plan, you now have the tools to support your personal resilience and increased freedom to engage in your best life.

If you're trying to work through Power-Ups and walking and have hit some stumbling blocks along the way, the next section addresses some common issues that people experience.

Expectations: Starting and Stopping

One of the biggest barriers to movement is how we compare ourselves to others or to our past selves, when we were younger or not sick or injured. When we get caught up in comparisons, we tend to focus on what we accomplish (or don't accomplish) rather than the fact that we made the effort, that we showed up.

A friend of Kristen's did cross-country running in college. After she graduated, she went to work at a bank, stopped running, and gained weight. She started running again and lost the weight, but when she changed jobs, time felt tight, and she quit running again and regained the weight. When she's not exercising, she manages her stress through bingeing on carbs. Recognizing that she was struggling with decreased energy and mental clarity and increased anxiety along with increased worry about the health consequences of the weight gain, she started running again and was able to recover the benefits. She went through this cycle a few times before she realized she was also stopping because she had become bored with running, so she started swimming, recovering all the benefits of exercise before stopping all movement activities again. When Kristen asked her why she was staying on this roller coaster, she explained that she didn't want to disappoint the friends she had made while engaging in each activity and was anxious about starting a new activity, so she would create "busyness" in her life as the excuse to fade out of the social groups. It was only the worry about health consequences that would push her into something new, and the cycle would start again. Kristen helped her create a plan that included developing a list of options so that she could more comfortably switch activities in a thought-out way. If you hit a plateau in your movement goals, or if you get bored with a single movement plan, it's okay to switch things up—what's important is to just keep showing up!

Another common challenge about movement and comparisons is the idea of continually getting better. One young man that Kristen was working with decided to do CrossFit. He went to a "box" (a popular term for a CrossFit gym) that emphasized safety, skill, and preventing injuries. He found that after being there for three months, his anxiety and depression were a lot better. He also loved that each month he was able to do more and more. The changes were measurable. "I improved 10 percent from last month and 60 percent from when I started." He wanted to continue to see these large improvements, but eventually the improvement curve began to flatten. Eventually, he came back to see Kristen because he was no longer doing well. When she asked what he was doing for movement, he said nothing: he had stopped because he didn't think it was worth the effort if he wasn't going to keep improving or being the best. Kristen wondered aloud if he had started CrossFit to be the best in the box or the state or to help with his energy and mental clarity. He looked at her sheepishly. This client had lost track of his positive feedback loop: Was it continued improvement or to feel better?

Does the cycle of starting and stopping sound familiar to you? What is your story, and what happened?

The Power of the Positive Feedback Loop

It's important to establish and recognize a positive feedback loop when starting a movement routine. When your reasons for exercising are the benefits that take weeks and months to realize, it's easier to come up with reasons for not following through. Many people find it much more empowering to focus on *feeling better now* as the motivating factor. Movement often gives you a slight bump in energy and mental clarity in the moment. If you really pay attention to that bump, it'll help you think, *I want more of that!* And little by little, that increase in energy helps you move more, which results in even larger gains. This is the positive feedback loop from movement.

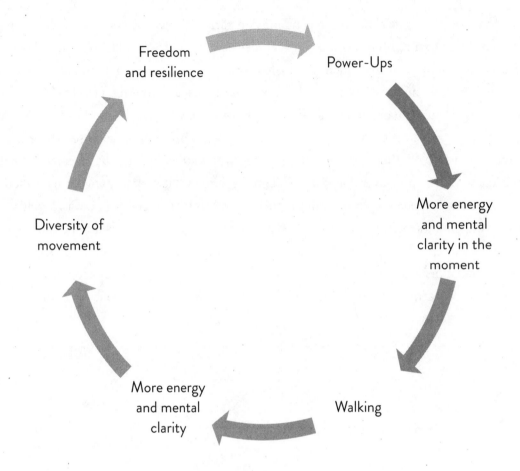

The Positive Feedback Loop from Movement

Moving your body is really about training the brain and body to work together more efficiently, which results in increased resilience to meet life's challenges. Look for the small wins first and, before you know it, you'll be navigating bigger challenges with more ease than you might have predicted.

BARRIERS FOR MOVEMENT

There are many reasons for avoiding movement: overly busy schedules, lack of childcare, and lack of supportive relationships, among others. "That we're lazy" is rarely true and often just the easy answer that keeps us from looking deeper. Many of us harbor past trauma, have experiences of feeling humiliated, were not encouraged to move, or did not have positive movement role models. Let's explore these a little deeper.

A History of Humiliation Around Moving Our Bodies

When Kristen starts discussing movement with her clients and she asks about their experiences, gym class inevitably comes up. Let's face it: most gym classes are taught by athletic people who prefer being around athletic people. If you didn't fit that mold, you may have felt left out. Some of us were also actively humiliated by the students or teachers. Kristen grew five inches in one summer during junior high school and, during that time, she didn't know where her feet and hands were, making gym class challenging.

Sometimes it's helpful to name what happened in the past that keeps us avoiding what we need or want in the now. Understanding that some of our self-perceptions are the result of past experiences can help us see that we have more control in our lives today to create a habit of movement that feels good to us. Is there anything that happened in the past that is now stopping you from moving your body?

A History of Trauma Creates Resistance to Moving

Another reason some people avoid moving their bodies is having a history of trauma (Oppizzi and Umberger 2018). During most traumatic events, our heart rates increase. Our bodies release adrenaline. We might find it hard to breathe. Somebody else might be in control of our bodies. There is often some overlap of physical response when we exercise and how we felt during the trauma. This can result in a resistance to having your heart rate increase, an avoidance of adrenaline, or a need to be in control and not be pushed into anything unfamiliar or uncomfortable. This all makes a lot of sense!

When we recognize that this might be the case, it can be helpful to talk about movement as a way to increase resilience to past trauma. Recognizing the root of your resistance to movement may help you decide that you don't want to continue letting the past determine your future. You may need to sit with this understanding for several months or even years before making a change. That's okay. Insight doesn't have to immediately change behavior, but we encourage you to lean into it and hold that truth until there is an internal need to change.

One day, a client with a history of sexual abuse as a child came into Kristen's office and said she was ready to stop letting her past limit what she does with her body. But every time she started an exercise program, the sensations caused by physical activity gave her flashbacks, anxiety, and insomnia. Kristen asked her if there was a place that she really liked to spend time other than home, a place that she had a positive association with, where she felt safe, and that was easy to get to. She thought about it and decided that the mall fit all those criteria.

This is the experiment she did: Kristen asked her to go to the mall as often as possible. The time she spent there would be bookmarked as her "practice time." She parked as far away as she felt comfortable and safe walking to the mall. Kristen encouraged her to walk around stores that she liked, not to buy something but to increase her enjoyment of being at the mall.

They worked on a practice plan that slowly increased the amount of movement she got with each visit to the mall. The second time she went, her client walked fast enough that she ran into the edge of the "I don't want to feel this" and then slowed down. Okay, there it was, and then she continued on to the mall more slowly and enjoyed her time there. The next time, she took a couple of steps into that feeling before slowing down, with the internal chant, "I'm excited to go to the mall." Over the course of a month or so, she got to the point where she was speed-walking to the mall.

Once she felt more comfortable and in control of the feeling, she started to expand this new skill to another location. She walked a path around a lake near her home. After she became more familiar with the path, she tried speed-walking and would just slow down if anything got triggered. After a time, she tried jogging, using an elliptical trainer, and swimming. She found that if she could anchor herself in the present moment by naming what she saw, heard, and felt, then she was fine. This gave her more confidence to challenge herself aerobically and in her personal life more generally.

Injury, Pain, or Fatigue: When Not to Move More

Kristen's patients are often surprised when she explicitly says, "Do not exercise…for now." Some of the reasons to put off adding movement include:

- Excessive fatigue, where a person's energy supply regularly maxes out at 5 out of 10.

- Regularly drinking more than two cups of coffee (or other caffeinated drinks) a day; this is a sign of fatigue.

- Chronic and persistent pain.

- Inability to prioritize feeding themselves; for example, moms of young babies can benefit from exercise, but if they can't prioritize feeding themselves regularly, adding movement can come later.

- Increased pain or fatigue with movement (meaning, there shouldn't be more fatigue or more pain the next day).

- Being told by a health care provider not to exercise.

If these things are true for you, that means you need to be getting some more support around your health before adding movement (see chapter 9). A great and safe way to start movement is with a physical therapist. If you have a body part that's in pain, remember the diversity of movement provided by different Power-Ups, which enables you to move uninjured body parts in safe doses.

Once you're inconsistently consistently adding movement to your routine, it's worth keeping in mind some minimum metrics for movement that will help you maintain independence throughout your life.

MINIMAL METRICS FOR MOVEMENT

Physical independence is so important to our self-identity. If your power supply limits activities essential for daily life because of fatigue, injury, disability, or disuse, you'll tend to have more anxiety because of fears around physical safety. Further, if your sense of isolation increases, worry, anxiety, and depression follow suit. Food, sleep, and movement are the three-legged stool that supports your power supply to ensure that you have the energy and mental clarity to navigate both the challenges and joys of your life with minimal worry and stress.

Consciously maintaining physical metrics for movement is one way to ensure continued freedom and hope. Some common minimal metrics are listed below to help you think through the basic skills that you may want to build or maintain. This list is also available online at http://www.newharbinger .com/46233.

Activity	I can do this.	I can't do this now, but I'll work toward this.
I can sit in a chair and stand up again without using my hands.		
I can comfortably walk for 10 minutes without being sore or fatigued the next day.		
I can comfortably walk for 30 minutes without being sore or fatigued the next day.		
I can comfortably walk for 60 minutes, without being sore or fatigued the next day.		
I am comfortable getting in and out of vehicles.		
I can carry two bags of groceries into my house.		
I can carry my laundry.		
I can bend to pick up a dropped item without losing my balance.		
I can walk up and down four flights of stairs without pain.		
I am comfortable walking through an airport with luggage.		
I can lift carry-on luggage into the overhead compartment comfortably and safely.		
I can sit on the floor and stand up again.		
I can bounce a ball off the floor and catch it 10 times.		
I can stand with my feet together and close my eyes for 30 seconds and not lose my balance.		
I don't limit my choices because of physical limitations.		
I can move without pain.		

What other movements are important to you to feel safe and confident when engaging in your life?

```
┌─────────────────────────────────────────────────────────────┐
│                                                             │
│                                                             │
│                                                             │
│                                                             │
│                                                             │
│                                                             │
│                                                             │
└─────────────────────────────────────────────────────────────┘
```

Keep this list in mind because sometimes these skills go away due to injury or changing priorities (for example, raising kids, developing your career, or time constraints).

CHAPTER SUMMARY

This chapter was all about physical activity and movement. In it, we reviewed reasons why people avoid physical activity and reasons why it's important not to do so. We also outlined three elements of a solid movement plan: seeding quick Power-Ups throughout your day to get you moving and combat anxiety and fatigue with quick energy boosts, building a sustainable routine of walking since walking is an incredibly helpful form of movement, and building in some more diverse movement activities that interest and engage you.

We suggested that starting with Power-Ups to improve energy in the moment is a good way to begin if you haven't been active recently. Building your ability to walk from 10 minutes up to an hour increases your freedom and independence, decreases your anxiety and fatigue, and improves your sleep quality. Honing the skill of starting something new and finding new activities that you enjoy doing will keep you emotionally engaged in movement. Finally, keeping track of what you physically need to be able to do in order to maintain independence and freedom to engage the world will help you maintain physical and mental resilience throughout your lifetime.

If you're unable to engage in Power-Ups or can't comfortably walk for 10 minutes, you might be struggling with a deeper source of fatigue. The next chapter provides tools to discuss your fatigue and search for underlying physiological causes with your health care provider.

## CHAPTER 9

Talking to Your Health Care Provider

Anxiety can have physical causes that can add to an already stressful situation, so it's worth ruling them out. But how do you ask your primary care provider to do more than just prescribe medications for anxiety and depression? How do you get them to rule out the physical causes of symptoms that might look like anxiety, depression, or fatigue? You have to know how to ask for what you want!

According to the National Institute of Mental Health (2017), in the United States, 46.6 million people live with some type of mental health issue. Prolonged fatigue is linked with anxiety and depression. However, all too often we assume that these symptoms are emotionally driven, without taking the time to rule out potential physical causes, such as hypoglycemia, low iron, or even possible drug interactions.

In part, this is because differentiating fatigue from anxiety and depression is hard to do, and those suffering often don't know what questions to ask. We always recommend that people begin by describing their symptoms to their primary health care providers as fatigue rather than labeling themselves as anxious or having depression. This way, providers might be more likely to consider the symptoms in and of themselves, rather than assuming the symptoms are emotional or psychological in nature. A good list to refer to for the overlap between physiological and emotional symptoms is the "global symptoms" list in chapter 1, "Snapshot of Anxiety."

It's important to be specific when you speak with your health care practitioner. Kristen spoke with a colleague who, for the last several years, was too fatigued to keep up with her housekeeping or participate in her hobbies and barely had enough bandwidth for her family. She had the basics covered nutritionally, was getting in some walking, and was sleeping nine hours a night, but she was still struggling. When she talked to her doctor, she felt her symptoms had been dismissed as middle age and menopause. Kristen suggested that she write down everything she was experiencing, including what her concerns were, make an appointment with her provider, and then simply read the letter aloud to the doctor. Kristen also advised her colleague to ask her provider to sign the letter, to indicate he'd received it, and to put it in her chart, even if the provider chose to do nothing about it.

Medical records are the property of the patient, the provider, and the organization, so everyone has the right to request that information be added to it—and this way, the full spectrum of symptoms Kristen's colleague was experiencing would be reflected in her medical records. When the colleague brought this list of symptoms to her doctor, he agreed to run the labs. The lab results indicated that Kristen's colleague indeed needed medication for a physiological condition, and once on the prescription, she began to feel normal again.

Fundamentally, each individual is responsible for their own health. Sometimes, this can be scary. We hope you're never in a position in which you have to fight for care you need and deserve or struggle to find answers that no professional seems willing or able to give you. But this reality can also be empowering. It can be a reminder that if you're not getting the care you want, you can educate yourself and increase your level of communication with your providers until the problem is addressed.

THE IMPORTANCE OF DIFFERENTIATING PHYSICAL FROM EMOTIONAL CAUSES OF FATIGUE, DEPRESSION, AND ANXIETY

A two-year study examined the case histories of 1,010 women with a diagnosis of iron deficiency (Blank et al. 2019). When these women initially asked their health care providers for help, due to feeling tired or fatigued, only 35 percent received the correct diagnosis of iron deficiency. The rest of the women (65 percent!) received a diagnosis of depression, burnout, anxiety, or chronic fatigue and received medication or psychotherapy. It was only later, when this second group of women did not improve with medication and/or therapy, that they had bloodwork done that correctly identified the iron deficiency. This correct diagnosis came months, and sometimes years, later.

What is particularly interesting is that this study also looked at the economic costs of missing a diagnosis of iron deficiency and calling it a mental health condition. In Swiss dollars (or Swiss francs, CHF), the annual direct medical costs were estimated to be CHF 78 million annually, and indirect costs were estimated to be CHF 33 million. These indirect costs are really important to these patients. This figure represents missed days of work and lower productivity; in their personal lives, it means not having the energy to connect with family and friends or to prepare food or to move their bodies. This is when anxiety and depression add to the fatigue caused by not having the nutrients to support an adequate power supply and feeling healthy. When you're so fatigued that you can't get the basics done, depression and anxiety can set in or get worse.

Often, only a complete blood count (CBC) lab is done to identify iron deficiency. For women specifically, iron deficiency is more common because of their menses and childbirth. The CBC is only a broad measure of iron and may not be truly screening for iron deficiencies. Because of this, Kristen encourages her clients to get additional iron labs that monitor iron, such as a ferritin test. While there is a cost for running these labs, the cost of treating fatigue, anxiety, and depression strictly as emotional symptoms is even higher.

There are a number of blood tests that can answer medical questions around fatigue. Below is a list of lab tests that Kristen finds helpful to rule out the physiological causes of fatigue, anxiety, and depression. These are labs that most primary care providers can and will run. While there are other labs that could be run, for the purposes of this book, we suggest starting with the basics that most people have access to through their primary care providers and that are covered by most insurance plans.

Labs that Assess Physiological Causes of Fatigue, Anxiety, and Depression

- **CBC (complete blood count)** rules out overt anemia, which causes fatigue.

- **Comprehensive metabolic panel** rules out liver and kidney problems and identifies issues with glucose regulation (prediabetes and diabetes directly affect brain function).

- **Lipid panel** is important in diagnosing cardiovascular disease. Additionally, when total cholesterol is below 150, suicidal ideation increases (Segoviano-Mendoza et al. 2018).

- **TSH (thyroid-stimulating hormone)** rules out hypothyroidism or hyperthyroidism. Low thyroid function can look like fatigue; elevated thyroid function can look like anxiety.

- **Ferritin (an iron marker)** levels below 50 correlate with increased fatigue, especially in women (Vaucher et al. 2012).

- **Hemoglobin A1C** is a marker for diabetes. Studies have shown that diabetes predicts depression and depression predicts diabetes: diabetes is a glucose control problem. As we have been discussing, anxiety can also be caused by glucose-regulation disorders.

- **CRP (C-reactive protein)** is an inflammation marker implicated in cardiovascular disease, diabetes, obesity, and depression. If elevated, you can experience fatigue.

- **Homocysteine (a vitamin B marker)** elevated levels indicate an increased risk of depression.

- **Vitamin D-25-OH** low levels can cause fatigue, depression, and musculoskeletal pain.

If you need to request that your primary care provider do any of these blood tests, we've created a sample letter that you can use to start this discussion (available in the appendix and for download at http://www.newharbinger.com/46233). Additionally, Kristen is always updating ways of identifying the physical causes of anxiety, fatigue, and depression and sharing them on our blog (http://www .kristenallott.com/blog).

If any of these test results come back abnormal or borderline, you likely have an underlying physical condition that is contributing to anxiety and fatigue, and can add to depression too, making it harder to manage. For good mental health, you want your physical body to have what it needs. Often, our bodies simply don't. And in today's medical system, where primary care providers typically have limited time with each patient, this letter can be used to remind them to consider anemia, thyroid dysfunction, inflammation, glucose control issues, and other conditions.

Luca Checks in with Her Primary Care Provider

For the last couple of months, Luca has been eating more frequent meals and snacks with protein. It took her a while to learn to be consistent with it and plan ahead. Even though it takes more time to do, Luca feels the effort is worth it because her bad anxiety and fatigue days aren't as bad. She's started making time for her hobby—knitting. Her low numbers on the energy scale in the Snapshot of Anxiety are 20 to 30 percent better on most days. Her symptoms of anxiety are a similar percentage lower. So, overall she is feeling better. But she wouldn't say that she's at her best. Luca decides to talk to her primary care provider about her fatigue. She makes an appointment with the nurse practitioner, Shawn, because she discovered that Shawn has more time than the medical doctor, and she seems to be more curious.

She takes the time to fill in the template letter with the labs list and fills out a new Snapshot of Anxiety Assessment. On the Snapshot worksheet, she adds her initial responses to the current ones in a different color to make it clear where she has improved and where she is still struggling. Additionally, she writes down what she typically is eating. Luca's a little nervous about being assertive about her care with Shawn. To make sure that there is no extra adrenaline in her system for the appointment, she eats half a turkey sandwich before she leaves and has two protein bars in her bag in case Shawn is running late.

At the medical office, she waits for Shawn in an examining room. Shawn enters and smiles. "Hi Luca. How can I help?" Luca responds, "I have been really working on my well-being over the last couple of months. I think I've underestimated how fatigued I am. I've been doing some reading on how labs can help identify some of the causes of fatigue. I was hoping that you could run these labs to make sure that everything is okay. Here's a list of my symptoms, my food intake, and the labs that I have read would be helpful. I'm most interested in TSH and ferritin. I have had a history of anemia, which has been better recently. As I understand, ferritin can still be low without anemia. Ferritin levels below 50 can cause fatigue in women, and I wonder if that's where my fatigue is coming from."

"Let me read through this for a moment. I appreciate that you came so prepared," replies Shawn. He looks up with concern and says, "I'm sorry that you are feeling so tired. I know in the past we have talked about anxiety. What if we consider an antidepressant medication?"

Luca's heart starts to beat faster. "Can we talk about the labs first? Do you have an issue with doing the labs?"

Shawn says, "No, I'm happy to do the labs. I just want to do something for you right now. We can do both."

Luca thinks about it for a minute. If she was not already feeling better from the changes in diet, sleep, and movement, she might consider the offer. But as she thinks about it, she knows that the really bad days are when she falls out of the new routine. Luca says, "You can write the prescription, but I might wait until I have the labs back to decide if I want to get it filled, if that is okay." Shawn says, "Absolutely!" Luca's heart slows. She silently gives herself a pat on the back for managing that moment and advocating for herself. Shawn gives her a slip with all the labs she requested and a script for medication. Luca realizes that it's true: all professionals offer the tools that they are most familiar with.

In two weeks, Luca is back in the office with Shawn. They go over the results. For this story, we are going to leave the results between the two of them. What's most important is that Luca helped Shawn be curious about her symptoms and engage in active problem solving. We hope you can do the same with your primary care provider, if that is the path you decide to take.

CHAPTER SUMMARY

Addressing the physiological causes of fatigue, anxiety, and depression can start with changes to food, sleep, and movement routines. However, it can also be important to rule out any underlying physical conditions that are contributing to your symptoms. This chapter outlined how to advocate for yourself and provided a list of which labs to request from your primary care provider so you can continue to move toward being your best.

Conclusion

It's now time to wrap up our journey together. Regardless of whether you read the workbook straight through without trying a single experiment or if you've been reading parts of this workbook for months or years, we are honored to have been part of your journey. Like all good personal journeys, it's worth considering the road that was traveled and to celebrate that you carried through on your path. One way to do this is to return to the Snapshot of Anxiety Assessment worksheet from chapter 1 (available at http://www.newharbinger.com/46233) to see if and how your symptoms have changed.

It's our wish that you'll carry with you the concept of hope. When you set a goal that you hope to achieve, focus on maintaining both waypower and willpower. The waypower is to create an experiment, or a path that can be followed, and when you run into an obstacle, to work to overcome it. This will require willpower, personal investment supported by brain-smart nutrition, to help you to continue to move forward toward your goal.

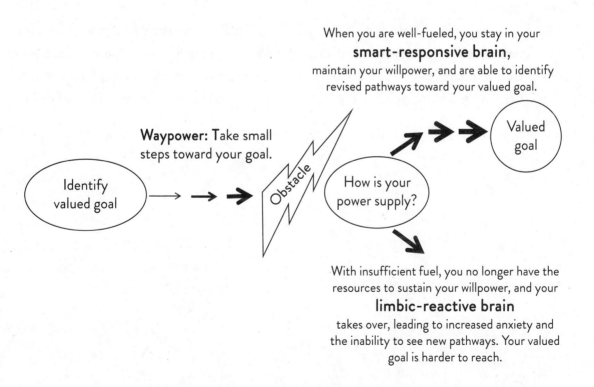

When you are well-fueled, you stay in your
smart-responsive brain,
maintain your willpower, and are able to identify
revised pathways toward your valued goal.

Waypower: Take small
steps toward your goal.

Obstacle

Identify
valued goal

How is your
power supply?

Valued
goal

With insufficient fuel, you no longer have the
resources to sustain your willpower, and your
limbic-reactive brain
takes over, leading to increased anxiety and
the inability to see new pathways. Your valued
goal is harder to reach.

How Well Can You Manage Your Willpower During Adversity?

Our hope in writing this workbook was to give you tools to reduce your anxiety and worry and increase your energy and mental clarity using food, sleep, movement, and appropriate diagnostic lab work. We hope these new tools will help you be at your best. Armed with this information, you can now:

- Watch and remedy the anxiety and fatigue that result from glucose fluctuation.

- Recognize when adrenaline causes you to switch away from your responsive-cortex brain into your reactive-limbic brain.

- Choose foods that can sustain your energy, or at least know that anxiety and worry will be creeping in a couple of hours after eating food without protein.

Perhaps you're also working to change your bedtime routine to sleep a little better. And we would be so happy if movement were beginning to be something you do to feel better right now! Movement is a kindness to yourself rather than an activity to be forced or thought of as a "should." Lastly, you have new information to help you have a constructive conversation with your health care provider to rule out the physiological dysfunctions that can mimic or exacerbate the symptoms of fatigue, anxiety, and depression.

This book is a beginning of where you can start. We will continue to share information with you at http://www.kristenallott.com. As you find success through experiments, we hope you share your experiences with your family, friends, and community. We offered this book as a way for all of us to help each other have less worry and anxiety and more energy and mental clarity so that we can all be at our best!

Appendix

CHAPTER 1: SNAPSHOT OF ANXIETY ASSESSMENT

Directions: <u>Part 1</u>: If your power supply drops below 5 during the active part of your day, give yourself a fatigue score of 10 points. If your power supply stays above 5, your fatigue score is 0. <u>Part 2</u>: If any part of the Brain-Body symptom description fits you, check the box and circle the part you relate to.

Part 1: Fatigue Score

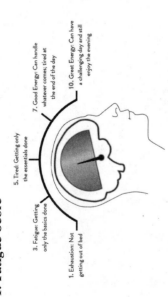

5. Tired: Getting only the essentials done

7. Good Energy: Can handle whatever comes; tired at the end of the day

3. Fatigue: Getting only the basics done

10. Great Energy: Can have a challenging day and still enjoy the evening

1. Exhaustion: Not getting out of bed

Take a moment to rate your power supply—or how much energy you feel you have—on a scale of 1 to 10, with 1 being minimal energy and 10 being solid energy throughout the day. If your power supply drops below 5 during the active part of your day, give yourself a fatigue score of 10 points. If your power supply stays above 5, your fatigue score is 0.

Circle Your Fatigue Score: 0   10

Part 2: Brain–Body Symptoms

BRAIN SYMPTOMS

☐ Flight emotions: agitation, nervousness, worry, anxiety, fear, panic

☐ Fight emotions: hyperfocused, defensive, negative, irritable, controlling, enraged

☐ Disappear emotions: withdrawn, depressed, crying, shut down

☐ Racing thoughts

☐ Negative thought patterns toward self; self-critical

☐ Emotional outbursts that are larger than necessary

☐ Doing old behaviors that you don't want to do again, such as eating sugar, drinking alcohol or using other addictive substances, or calling people that are not helpful

☐ Fear of dying, suicidal thoughts, confusion, abnormal behavior— *If you check this box, please ask for help or call 911.*

BODY SYMPTOMS

☐ Shaky or trembling hands

☐ Heart palpitations, racing heart rate

☐ Shortness of breath

☐ Pale skin, cold hands and feet

☐ Shakiness, vibrating body, physically agitated, or fidgety

☐ Hungry, craving sugar, sweets, or carbohydrates (breads, pasta, candy)

☐ Nausea

☐ Not hungry for meals or not able to eat

☐ Sweating

☐ Dizziness

☐ Vertigo

☐ Visual disturbance

☐ Extreme fatigue

☐ Seizures or loss of consciousness

Total number of boxes checked: [   ] / 22

CHAPTER 1: SNAPSHOT OF ANXIETY ASSESSMENT

Directions: Part 3: Use the rating scale to answer the Global Symptoms questions. Add the totals from each column to get your score. Skip questions that don't apply to you. Part 4: Write in the totals from Parts 1, 2, and 3 to get your Snapshot of Anxiety Score

Part 3: Global Symptoms: The Physiological Process That Increases Anxiety Can also Increase Other Symptoms

Please rate these symptoms	Not at all	Some days	Most days	Nearly every day
Fatigue	0	1	2	3
Afternoon fatigue	0	1	2	3
Moodiness, including emotions of anxiety, irritation, agitation, and sadness	0	1	2	3
Lack of mental clarity	0	1	2	3
Morning insomnia/waking too early	0	1	2	3
Inability to wake up in morning	0	1	2	3
PTSD nightmares	0	1	2	3
Brain fog/Harder to think	0	1	2	3
Physical pain for any cause	0	1	2	3
Distraction and/or ADHD symptoms	0	1	2	3
Dysregulated bowel symptoms (constipations, diarrhea, bloating)	0	1	2	3
Sugar/carbohydrate cravings	0	1	2	3
The use alcohol or other substances to regulate your emotions and symptoms	0	1	2	3
Subtotal Score:				
Total Score (add the scores from the 4 columns above):				

Part 4: Snapshot of Anxiety Assessment Score

	Points
From Part 1: Fatigue Score	
From Part 2: Brain–Body Symptoms total points	
From Part 3: Global Symptoms total points from all columns	
Snapshot of Anxiety Score:	

You might be curious about how to interpret your final score. However, when it comes to the Snapshot of Anxiety, there isn't a standard total. Instead, you'll be using the score to see if your ratings for each category improve when you do experiments.

Identify what's most important to you about reducing anxiety:

Benefits	Not important	Somewhat important	Mostly important	Very important
Feel better				
Better sleep				
More confident				
More at ease with yourself				
Willing to try new things				
Better connections and/or boundaries with friends and family				
Better able to take care of projects important to you				
Other:				

What Impacts Anxiety	Day 1 Date:	Day 2 Date:	Day 3 Date:
	What's going on?	What's going on?	What's going on?
Time of day			
Power Supply (1-10)			
ANXIETY LEVEL — HIGH: 10, 9, 8, 7			
ANXIETY LEVEL — MED: 6, 5, 4			
ANXIETY LEVEL — LOW: 3, 2, 1			
Anxiety Accelerators (Caffeine, Alcohol, Sugary Foods, Screen Time, Stressful Day)			
Daily Practices:			
What did you eat (meal or snack)? (Protein, Carb, Veggie/Fiber, Fat)			
☑ Movement/Physical Activity			
☑ Safe, Supportive Connections			
Resiliency Factors (Mindfulness, Quiet Time, Time Outside, Spiritual Practice, Journaling)			
# of hours of sleep the night before			
Other Notes			

Brain diagram labels: 1. Fine 3. Low 5. Medium 7. High 10. Panic Attack/Total Shutdown

CHAPTER 3: I NEED HELP NOW!

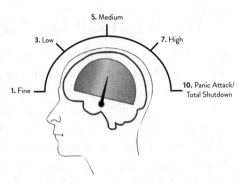

This handout summarizes some key interventions to help you feel better now. Consider the questions below and take action as needed. When you're feeling on the edge and having a hard time with acute anxiety and worry, it's hard to remember what you can do in the moment to help yourself. Keep this tip sheet handy so you can refer to it as needed.

If you are experiencing any of the below, try a **Lizard Brain Treat**! Even though you may not feel hungry, fueling your brain will help you reduce your anxiety and symptoms.

1. Are you having a panic attack?

2. Are you uncomfortably anxious or irritated?

3. Are you waking at 3 in the morning, with your mind racing?

4. Are you overly or underly emotional for the situation?

5. Have you not eaten for more than 3 hours?

6. Do you want to feel better in 10–15 minutes?

Lizard Brain Treat

A Lizard Brain Treat is a snack of sugar (a quick fuel) and protein (a longer-lasting fuel). You want the quick fuel to get to your brain almost immediately, which will start to reduce the adrenaline causing you to be in your reactive-limbic brain (or lizard brain). Following this with protein extends the amount of time you're in your responsive-cortex brain, before needing to refuel. Choose one quick fuel and one protein from the lists below—or from your favorite foods.

Ideas for Quick Fuels:	**Ideas for Protein:**
¼ cup of juice	¼ cup of nuts
1 piece of hard candy	A stick of jerky
¼ cup of soda	¼ cup of cottage cheese
Honey stick	2 tbsp of peanut (or other nut) butter
1 tbsp of jelly	

> **Combined sources work too (as long as they aren't sugar-free)!**
> - ½ cup of a protein shake
> - Protein bar
> - ½ PB&J sandwich

☑ **Generally speaking, your anxiety will drop by 10–20% within 10–15 minutes.**

What other things help you feel better?

BEING AT YOUR BEST DURING HIGH-STAKES EVENTS

Are you going to an event that you know will make you feel uncomfortable or anxious? Our natural tendency is to not eat in these situations, which only increases the hormone-signaling that this is a stressful event, releasing more adrenaline. To stay in the responsive-cortex brain—and out of the reactive-limbic brain (or lizard brain)—it's helpful to make sure that your brain and body have enough fuel to manage the high-stakes event.

By eating food that contains both carbohydrates and a sufficient amount of protein (as well as healthy fat and some fiber), your brain will be fueled for 2–4 hours. Getting around 20 grams of protein in a meal will last you longer. (*Note: eating more than 20 grams of protein at one time does not extend this benefit.*)

Examples of high-stakes events:

→ Any situation where you want to be at your best

→ Being around people that stress you out

→ Doing something new

→ Being around highly emotional people

→ Family events

→ Work-related social events

→ Job interviews

→ Test taking

→ Going to therapy

→ Public speaking

→ Going to court

Some examples of high-protein snacks and meals:

Animal-based

- Cottage cheese or Greek yogurt
- Protein shakes and bars (whey, egg, bone broth powders)
- A few slices of deli meat such as chicken or turkey with carrots or pita bread
- Deli salad with chicken or turkey
- Teriyaki chicken kabobs
- Hard-boiled eggs with carrots or pita bread
- Chicken sandwich
- Tacos or burritos (with meat)

Plant-based

- Hummus with carrots, celery, or pita bread
- Baba ghanoush with corn chips
- Nut butter sandwich
- Nut butter with apple slices
- Protein shakes and bars (rice, pea, soy protein powders)
- Tofu salads, sandwiches, or wraps
- Bag of mixed, non-roasted nuts (hazelnuts, walnuts, almonds, cashews)
- Tacos or burritos (with beans or tofu)

Here are some visual clues to help you get enough protein:

- 3 oz meat = a deck of playing cards
- 1 c yogurt = a hand holding a tennis ball
- ½ c cooked grain = a small fist

- 1 oz cheese = a thumb
- 1 oz nuts = a golf ball
- 1 tbsp nut butter or nuts = a silver dollar

CHAPTER 7: EXPERIMENTS FOR BETTER SLEEP

Sleep is essential for clear thinking and vibrant energy. As discussed in chapter 7, there are several night-time disturbances made worse by glucose-regulation problems: early-morning waking, nightmares and PTSD night terrors, oversleeping, not being functional in the morning, and not being hungry for breakfast. We encourage you to try the following experiments. Using the Snapshot of Anxiety Assessement before and after an experiment will help you recognize how sleeping better reduces anxiety, worry, and fatigue.

Remember: it can take 10–14 days to see the impact of experiments for improving sleep.

Fuel Your Brain Before Sleep

Try adding a protein snack (7–10 grams) shortly before going to bed. This could be a couple slices of turkey, a ¼ cup of cottage cheese or Greek yogurt, or a ¼ cup of nuts. See the protein chart in chapter 4 for more ideas.

This will help reduce sleep disturbances in the middle of the night caused by running out of fuel for your brain to do its important tasks while you sleep.

Have a Lizard Brain Treat

A Lizard Brain Treat is a ¼ cup of (100%) juice plus a handful (~¼ cup) of nuts (or equivalent protein). Remember the physiology? The juice provides the quick fuel which will help you fall back asleep faster, and the nuts provide protein, the longer-lasting fuel which will help you stay asleep longer. For this experiment, keep your Lizard Brain Treat near your bed for easy access.

This will help you fall back asleep faster if you wake up and can't stop your racing thoughts, or wake from a nightmare or PTSD night terror.

Eat Breakfast

If you wake up and aren't hungry for breakfast, have a hard time functioning, or feel numb or detached, you likely already have adrenaline in your system. You may not feel hungry, but your brain and body need fuel! Start with a ¼ cup of juice shortly after waking, followed by a balanced breakfast (protein, healthy carbs, healthy fat, and fiber), within 20–30 minutes. See chapter 6 for breakfast ideas.

This will help you function better in the mornings, and will also help reduce afternoon fatigue and sugar cravings.

Routines for Bed to Improve Sleep

A lack of sleep routine can create fatigue, mental health problems, and physical health problems such as obesity and diabetes. Decide when you want to be in bed and when you want to get up, and then try some of the following to help you follow through with this intention:

- Reduce the amount of high-carbohydrate foods (sweets, chips, alcohol) you eat before bed.

- Avoid scary or high-adrenaline TV shows and books before bed.

- Don't use screens (phones, tablets, TVs) within 30 minutes of going to bed.

- Pay attention to your sleep clock (chapter 7)—When do you feel a little sleepy in the evenings? When do you feel it again? Learning your body's rhythms will help you work with your physiology.

- Use your bed only for sleep and sex.

This will help you function better in the mornings, and will also help reduce afternoon fatigue and sugar cravings (although the first few days might be a little more difficult).

CHAPTER 7: EXPERIMENTS FOR FALLING ASLEEP

What are the sleep issues you want to address?

What experiment are you doing?

Use the below table to keep track of whatever information will help you stay on track with your experiment:

Date														
Day	1	2	3	4	5	6	7	8	9	10	11	12	13	14
Last meal before sleep (time)														
Last refined carb/alcohol (time)														
Protein snack before bed (Y/N)														
Early-morning Lizard Brain Treat (Y/N)														
Sleep Clock (time):														
1st Sleep Bell														
2nd Sleep Bell														
3rd Sleep Bell														
Other notes: *Slept great? Didn't sleep so well? Make some notes about what might have contributed to this, so you can begin to recognize patterns.*														

CHAPTER 8: EXPERIMENTS WITH MOVEMENT TO IMPROVE ENERGY AND MENTAL CLARITY

Element 1: Power-Ups. Are you willing to try something for just 30 seconds? Until people are able to feel the effect in their own bodies, some may dismiss this as "not enough to be worth doing."

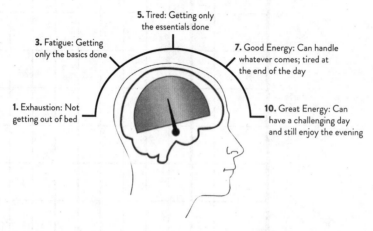

1. Check in and rate your energy level at this moment, using the Power Supply scale.

   _____

2. Now stand up. Choose one of the Power-Up movements that you will do four times.

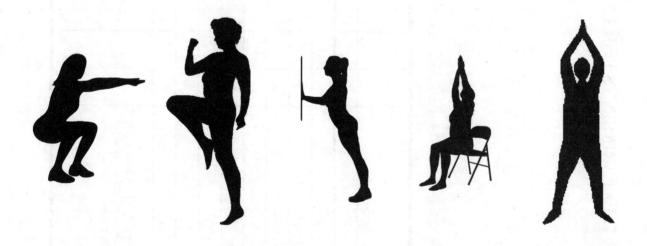

☐ **Chair squats** – have a chair behind you and sit down as though you are going to take a seat. Just as the chair touches you, stand back up;

☐ **March in place** – with your knees coming up as high as it is comfortable;

☐ **Wall push-ups** – place your hands on a wall with your feet about arm's length away from the wall; bend your arms until your nose is near the wall or you think is close enough; push back out to an upright position;

☐ **Overhead hand clap** – raise both arms in the air and bring your hands together comfortably over your head. Clap your hands together if that sounds like fun.

Remember one of these, just four times.

3.   Sit back down and rerate your energy level. _____

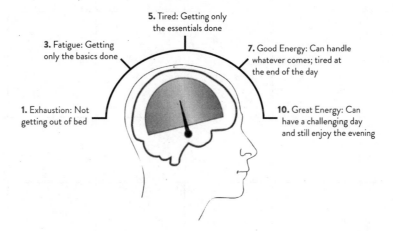

5. Tired: Getting only the essentials done

3. Fatigue: Getting only the basics done

7. Good Energy: Can handle whatever comes; tired at the end of the day

1. Exhaustion: Not getting out of bed

10. Great Energy: Can have a challenging day and still enjoy the evening

How to build a Power-Up program. Find moments throughout the day that you can insert a Power-Up. Experiment with the number of times you can comfortably do the movement. What happens if you do six instead of four? What happens if you do 10? What happens if you do them four, five times in the same day? Be playful. Where can you place these Power-Ups to improve your day? Before a meeting? After a meeting? Before picking up the kids from school? Before or after you get in or out of a car? In the bathroom? When you get off the couch from watching TV? Once you get into the routine of adding Power-Ups throughout the day, add variety in the type of Power-Ups you do. We recommend going to YouTube and trying these search terms: chair yoga, desk exercises or core exercises. Keep notes on which you did, how many times, and your energy level before and after.

Date	Time	Energy Level	Power-Up	# Reps	Energy Level	Notes

Element 2: Walking. For the walking experiment, we're going to take you through a few questions to help you shape your own experiment because everyone is different. For this experiment, your goal is to have more energy and mental clarity and less worry and anxiety. Other benefits will come with time, but this is a good starting point.

1. Rate your energy level: _____   Rate your anxiety range during the week: _____

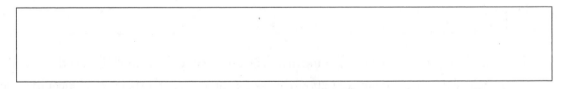

What's your power supply?   What's your anxiety level?

2. How long or far can you comfortably walk right now, without causing discomfort in any way? Can you already walk for 10 minutes? If not, set a distance goal: to a mailbox, the corner, a loop around the house, or whatever other mark feels right.

3. What time, or times, will you add this activity into your day? _____
    Give yourself permission for it to end up being inconsistently consistent.

4. How many times are you willing to commit to the experiment?_____
    Our recommendation is to hit 30 days within a 45-day period. However, that might not be realistic in your life. Please make a realistic goal for yourself. You don't have to wait for a "free" 45-day period! Just extend the 45 days to however long you need in order to hit the mark of walking 30 separate times.

5. How will you monitor the number of times you walk? We have found that, for many people, marking it in a calendar isn't effective. Consider creating a visually tangible system, such as an "I did it" vase.

6. What will you do when you go out for a walk, to keep yourself interested in the activity?

You're ready to begin! Consider sharing your reflections with family members, friends, or a therapist, or be sure to share with yourself through journaling or by naming to yourself what you remember about the walk at the end of the day. This is a good way to reinforce the activity of walking.

7. Now that you're into the experiment... Have you gone for a walk 10–20 times yet? Some people will notice differences in how they feel right away, and others take longer to notice the effects. Both are okay! The important thing is to keep checking in with yourself throughout the experiment. Remember not to make decisions about the utility of the experiment until the end, because you don't know if how you feel will change over time. Have you noticed changes in how you feel in your body and mind since you began the experiment? Have you noticed if you can walk more comfortably, or further within the same time frame? Did you stay with your original time frame, or were there times you walked for longer, or shorter?

8.   You did it – you completed 30 days of walking! Congratulations! What happened over the course of the experiment? Let's check back in with the questions you answered at the beginning.

a.   Rate your power supply: _____   Rate your anxiety range during the week: _____

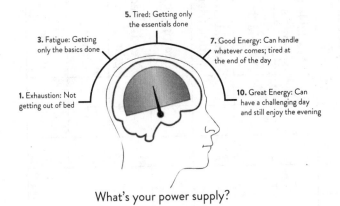

What's your power supply?

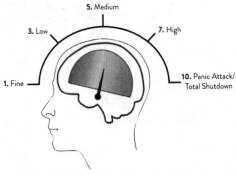

What's your anxiety level?

b.   How long or far can you comfortably walk right now, without causing discomfort in any way? Has this changed since the beginning of the experiment?

_____

c.   What else have you noticed that has changed since you started walking more regularly? Common things are that Power-Ups are easier, anxiety is lower, sleep is better, and self-confidence may have improved. Remember that these are just some of the things that some people notice—it's okay if what you experience is different.

d.   Do you plan to continue a practice of walking? _____

9.   Now that you've completed this experiment in walking, what's your next experiment? Hopefully, walking in an inconsistently consistent way has increased your energy and mental clarity and reduced your anxiety and worry. One option is to do another experiment that changes the duration, distance, or frequency that you walk.

Element 3: Adding Diversity. Finding movement activities that are easily accessible is easier if you can create a list of what is available near you.

Activities Chart	Convenience (location)	Convenience (timing)	Available every day	Available some days	Available in specific seasons	Would do alone	Would do only with a friend	Multiple benefits	Needs special gear	Other	Rank
1.											
2.											
3.											
4.											
5.											
6.											
7.											
8.											
9.											
10.											
11.											
12.											
13.											
14.											
15.											
16.											
17.											
18.											
19.											
20.											

CHAPTER 9. EXAMPLE LETTER TO YOUR PRIMARY CARE PROVIDER

Fill out (or modify) the following letter and take it to your primary care provider.

Dear _____,

I would like you to rule out physical causes of the symptoms I'm experiencing (all that apply are checked):

☐ Fatigue   ☐ Constipation

☐ Palpitations   ☐ Diarrhea

☐ Insomnia, early-morning waking   ☐ Alternating constipation and diarrhea

☐ Insomnia, difficulty falling asleep   ☐ Weight loss

☐ Heavy menstrual bleeding   ☐ Restless legs

☐ Headaches   ☐ Skin conditions, acne, eczema, psoriasis

☐ Weight gain   ☐ Physical pain in the following places:

                                                             _____

Other symptoms:

I understand that the *Diagnostic and Statistical Manual of Mental Disorders* (DSM-5) requires that a full medical exam (physical exam and blood panel) be performed to screen for preexisting medical conditions before any mental health diagnosis is made.

It is my understanding that the following labs help rule out fatigue:

- **CBC (complete blood count)** rules out overt anemia, which causes fatigue.

- **Comprehensive metabolic panel** rules out liver and kidney problems and identifies issues with glucose regulation (prediabetes and diabetes directly affect brain function).

- **Lipid panel** is important in diagnosing cardiovascular disease. Additionally, when total cholesterol is below 150, suicidal ideation increases (Segoviano-Mendoza et al. 2018).

- **TSH (thyroid-stimulating hormone)** rules out hypothyroidism or hyperthyroidism. Low thyroid function can look like fatigue; elevated thyroid function can look like anxiety.

- **Ferritin (an iron marker)** levels below 50 correlate with increased fatigue, especially in women (Vaucher et al. 2012).

- **Hemoglobin A1C** is a marker for diabetes. Studies have shown that diabetes predicts depression and depression predicts diabetes: diabetes is a glucose control problem. As we have been discussing, anxiety can also be caused by glucose-regulation disorders.

- **CRP (C-reactive protein)** is an inflammation marker implicated in cardiovascular disease, diabetes, obesity, and depression. If elevated, you can experience fatigue.

- **Homocysteine (a vitamin B marker)** elevated levels indicate an increased risk of depression.

- **Vitamin D-25-OH** low levels can cause fatigue, depression, and musculoskeletal pain .

I would appreciate it if you would order these tests. Additionally, if there are any labs that you are unable to request, please include a signed note in my chart that I requested them.

Sincerely,

Worksheets and Additional Resources

If you need extra copies of the worksheets, or prefer not to write in this workbook, you can download them, as well as additional resources at http://www.newharbinger.com/46233 and at https://www.kristenallott.com.

Chapter 1: Snapshot of Anxiety Assessment

Chapter 2: What Impacts Anxiety

Chapter 3: I Need Help Now!

Chapter 3: Being at Your Best for High-Stakes Events

Chapter 4: Three-Day Protein Experiment Tracking Worksheet

Chapter 5: Steps for Understanding Food Labels/Food Label Comparison Worksheet

Chapter 6: Mix and Match Food Choices and Preparation Styles

Chapter 6: Emergency Food Plan

Chapter 7: Experiments for Better Sleep

Chapter 7: Experiments for Falling Asleep

Chapter 8: Experiments with Movement to Improve Energy and Mental Clarity

Chapter 9: Example Letter to Your Primary Care Provider

Bibliography

Alkadhi, Karim, Munder Zagaar, Ibrahim Alhaider, Samina Salim, and Abdulaziz Aleisa. 2013. "Neurobiological Consequences of Sleep Deprivation." *Current Neuropharmacology* 11 (3): 231–249.

American Psychiatric Association. 2013. *Diagnostic and Statistical Manual of Mental Disorders, 5th Edition (DSM-5)*. Washington, DC: APA Publishing.

Arthur, C. K., and J. P. Isbister. 1987. "Iron Deficiency: Misunderstood, Misdiagnosed, and Mistreated." *Drugs* 33 (2): 171–182.

Blank, Patricia R., Yuki Tomonaga, Thomas D. Szucs, and Matthias Schwenkglenks. 2019. "Economic Burden of Symptomatic Iron Deficiency—A Survey Among Swiss Women." *BMC Women's Health* 19 (1): 39.

Booth, Frank W., Christian K. Roberts, and Matthew J. Laye. 2012. "Lack of Exercise Is a Major Cause of Chronic Diseases." *Comprehensive Physiology* 2 (2): 1143–1211.

Chau, Josephine Y., Anne C. Grunseit, Tien Chey, Emmanuel Stamatakis, Wendy J. Brown, Charles E. Matthews, Adrian E. Bauman, and Hidde P. van der Ploeg. 2013. "Daily Sitting Time and All-Cause Mortality: A Meta-Analysis." *PLoS One* 8 (11): e80000.

Consensus Conference Panel, Nathaniel F. Watson, M. Safwan Badr, Gregory Belenky, Donald L. Bliwise, Orfeu M. Buxton, et al. 2015. "Joint Consensus Statement of the American Academy of Sleep Medicine and Sleep Research Society on the Recommended Amount of Sleep for a Healthy Adult: Methodology and Discussion." *Sleep* 38 (8): 1161–1183; 11 (8): 931–952.

Deschênes, Sonya S., Rachel J. Burns, and Norbert Schmitz. 2018. "Comorbid Depressive and Anxiety Symptoms and the Risk of Type 2 Diabetes: Findings from the Lifelines Cohort Study." *Journal of Affective Disorders* 238 (October): 24–31.

Dipnall, Joanna F., Julie A. Pasco, Denny Meyer, Michael Berk, Lana J. Williams, Seetal Dodd, and Felice N. Jacka. 2015. "The Association Between Dietary Patterns, Diabetes, and Depression." *Journal of Affective Disorders* 174 (March): 215–224.

Dregan, A., and M. C. Gulliford. 2013. "Leisure-Time Physical Activity over the Life Course and Cognitive Functioning in Late Mid-Adult Years: A Cohort-Based Investigation." *Psychological Medicine* 43 (11): 2447–2458.

Edwards, Meghan K., and Paul D. Loprinzi. 2018. "Experimental Effects of Brief, Single Bouts of Walking and Meditation on Mood Profile in Young Adults." *Health Promotion Perspectives* 8 (3): 171–178.

Edwards, Meghan K., and Paul D. Loprinzi. 2019. "Affective Responses to Acute Bouts of Aerobic Exercise, Mindfulness Meditation, and Combinations of Exercise and Meditation: A Randomized Controlled Intervention." *Psychological Reports* 122 (2): 465–484.

Engle-Friedman, Mindy. 2014. "The Effects of Sleep Loss on Capacity and Effort." *Sleep Science* 7 (4): 213–224.

Fernandez-Mendoza, Julio, and Alexandros N. Vgontzas. 2013. "Insomnia and Its Impact on Physical and Mental Health." *Current Psychiatry Reports* 15 (12): 418.

Firth, Joseph, Wolfgang Marx, Sarah Dash, Rebekah Carney, Scott B. Teasdale, Marco Solmi, et al. 2019. "The Effects of Dietary Improvement on Symptoms of Depression and Anxiety: A Meta-Analysis of Randomized Controlled Trials." *Psychosomatic Medicine* 81 (3): 265–280.

Garatachea, Nuria, Helios Pareja-Galeano, Fabian Sanchis-Gomar, Alejandro Santos-Lozano, Carmen Fiuza-Luces, María Morán, et al. 2015. "Exercise Attenuates the Major Hallmarks of Aging." *Rejuvenation Research* 18 (1): 57–89.

Goldstein-Piekarski, Andrea N., Stephanie M. Greer, Jared M. Saletin, and Matthew P. Walker. 2015. "Sleep Deprivation Impairs the Human Central and Peripheral Nervous System Discrimination of Social Threat." *The Journal of Neuroscience: The Official Journal of the Society for Neuroscience* 35 (28): 10135–10145.

Goldstein-Piekarski, Andrea N., Stephanie M. Greer, Jared M. Saletin, Allison G. Harvey, Leanne M. Williams, and Matthew P. Walker. 2017. "Sex, Sleep Deprivation, and the Anxious Brain." *Journal of Cognitive Neuroscience* 30 (4): 565–578.

Gwinn, Casey, and Chan M. Hellman. 2019. *HOPE Rising: How the Science of HOPE Can Change Your Life.* New York: Morgan James Publishing.

Hoare, Erin, Karen Milton, Charlie Foster, and Steven Allender. 2017. "Depression, Psychological Distress and Internet Use Among Community-Based Australian Adolescents: A Cross-Sectional Study." *BMC Public Health* 17 (1): 365.

Honn, K. A., J. M. Hinson, P. Whitney, and H. P. A. Van Dongen. 2019. "Cognitive Flexibility: A Distinct Element of Performance Impairment Due to Sleep Deprivation." *Accident Analysis & Prevention* 126 (May): 191–197.

Hrafnkelsdottir, Soffia M., Robert J. Brychta, Vaka Rognvaldsdottir, Sunna Gestsdottir, Kong Y. Chen, Erlingur Johannsson, et al. 2018. "Less Screen Time and More Frequent Vigorous Physical Activity Is Associated with Lower Risk of Reporting Negative Mental Health Symptoms Among Icelandic Adolescents." *PLoS One* 13 (4): e0196286.

Irwin, Michael R., Richard Olmstead, and Judith E. Carroll. 2016. "Sleep Disturbance, Sleep Duration, and Inflammation: A Systematic Review and Meta-Analysis of Cohort Studies and Experimental Sleep Deprivation." *Biological Psychiatry* 80 (1): 40–52.

Jacka, Felice N., Julie A. Pasco, Arnstein Mykletun, Lana J. Williams, Allison M. Hodge, Sharleen Linette O'Reilly, et al. 2010. "Association of Western and Traditional Diets with Depression and Anxiety in Women." *American Journal of Psychiatry* 167 (3): 305–311.

Jacka, Felice N., Adrienne O'Neil, Rachelle Opie, Catherine Itsiopoulos, Sue Cotton, Mohammedreza Mohebbi, et al. 2017. "A Randomised Controlled Trial of Dietary Improvement for Adults with Major Depression (the 'SMILES' Trial)." *BMC Medicine* 15 (1): 23.

Jacka, Felice N., Adrienne O'Neil, Catherine Itsiopoulos, Rachelle Opie, Sue Cotton, Mohammadreza Mohebbi, et al. 2018. "The SMILES Trial: An Important First Step." *BMC Medicine* 16 (1): 237.

Kandel, Eric R., James Harris Schwartz, and Thomas M. Jessell. 2000. *Principles of Neural Science.* Fourth Edition. New York: McGraw-Hill, Health Professions Division.

Kandola, Aaron, Davy Vancampfort, Matthew Herring, Amanda Rebar, Mats Hallgren, Joseph Firth, and Brendon Stubbs. 2018. "Moving to Beat Anxiety: Epidemiology and Therapeutic Issues with Physical Activity for Anxiety." *Current Psychiatry Reports* 20 (8): 63.

Lydon, David M., Nilam Ram, David E. Conroy, Aaron L. Pincus, Charles F. Geier, and Jennifer L. Maggs. 2016. "The Within-Person Association Between Alcohol Use and Sleep Duration and Quality *in Situ*: An Experience Sampling Study." *Addictive Behaviors* 61: 68–73.

Madhav, K. C., Shardulendra Prasad Sherchand, and Samendra Sherchan. 2017. "Association Between Screen Time and Depression Among US Adults." *Preventive Medicine Reports* 8 (December): 67–71.

Martin, Elizabeth I., Kerry J. Ressler, Elisabeth Binder, and Charles B. Nemeroff. 2009. "The Neurobiology of Anxiety Disorders: Brain Imaging, Genetics, and Psychoneuroendocrinology." *The Psychiatric Clinics of North America* 32 (3): 549–575.

McCarthy, Michael J., and David K. Welsh. 2012. "Cellular Circadian Clocks in Mood Disorders." *Journal of Biological Rhythms* 27 (5): 339–352.

Nabi, Hermann, Murielle Bochud, Jennifer Glaus, Aurélie M. Lasserre, Gérard Waeber, Peter Vollenweider, and Martin Preisig. 2013. "Association of Serum Homocysteine with Major Depressive Disorder: Results from a Large Population-Based Study." *Psychoneuroendocrinology* 38 (10): 2309–2318.

National Institute of Mental Health. 2017. "Mental Illness." National Institute of Mental Health. Accessed August 7, 2020. https://www.nimh.nih.gov/health/statistics/mental-illness.shtml.

National Sleep Foundation. February 2, 2015. "National Sleep Foundation Recommends New Sleep Times." Accessed August 7, 2019. http://www.sleepfoundation.org/press-release/national-sleep-foundation -recommends-new-sleep-times..

Opie, Rachelle S., Adrienne O'Neil, Catherine Itsiopoulos, and Felice N. Jacka. 2015. "The Impact of Whole-of-Diet Interventions on Depression and Anxiety: A Systematic Review of Randomised Controlled Trials." *Public Health Nutrition* 18 (11): 2074–2093.

Oppizzi, Lauren M., and Reba Umberger. 2018. "The Effect of Physical Activity on PTSD." *Issues in Mental Health Nursing* 39 (2): 179–187.

Parthasarathy, Sairam, Mary A. Carskadon, Girardin Jean-Louis, Judith Owens, Adam Bramoweth, Daniel Combs, et al. 2016. "Implementation of Sleep and Circadian Science: Recommendations from the Sleep Research Society and National Institutes of Health Workshop." *Sleep* 39 (12): 2061–2075.

Paruthi, Shalini, Lee J. Brooks, Carolyn D'Ambrosio, Wendy A. Hall, Suresh Kotagal, Robin M. Lloyd, et al. 2016. "Recommended Amount of Sleep for Pediatric Populations: A Consensus Statement of the American Academy of Sleep Medicine." *Journal of Clinical Sleep Medicine* 12 (6): 785–786.

Ratey, John J., and Eric. Hagerman. 2008. *Spark: The Revolutionary New Science of Exercise and the Brain*. New York: Little, Brown Spark.

Richardson, Caroline R., Guy Faulkner, Judith McDevitt, Gary S. Skrinar, Dori S. Hutchinson, and John D. Piette. 2005. "Integrating Physical Activity into Mental Health Services for Persons with Serious Mental Illness." *Psychiatric Services* 56 (3): 324–331.

Schmitt, Karen, Edith Holsboer-Trachsler, and Anne Eckert. 2016. "BDNF in Sleep, Insomnia, and Sleep Deprivation." *Annals of Medicine* 48 (1–2): 42–51.

Segoviano-Mendoza, Marcela, Manuel Cárdenas-de la Cruz, José Salas-Pacheco, Fernando Vázquez-Alaniz, Osmel La Llave-León, Francisco Castellanos-Juárez, et al. 2018. "Hypocholesterolemia Is an Independent Risk Factor for Depression Disorder and Suicide Attempt in Northern Mexican Population." *BMC Psychiatry* 18 (1): 7.

Siegel, Daniel J. 2010. *Mindsight: The New Science of Personal Transformation*. New York: Bantam Books.

Simon, Eti Ben, Noga Oren, Haggai Sharon, Adi Kirschner, Noam Goldway, Hadas Okon-Singer, et al. 2015. "Losing Neutrality: The Neural Basis of Impaired Emotional Control without Sleep." *The Journal of Neuroscience: The Official Journal of the Society for Neuroscience* 35 (38): 13194–13205.

Skonieczna-Żydecka, Karolina, Wojciech Marlicz, Agata Misera, Anastasios Koulaouzidis, and Igor Łoniewski. 2018. "Microbiome—The Missing Link in the Gut-Brain Axis: Focus on Its Role in Gastrointestinal and Mental Health." Journal of Clinical Medicine 7(12), 521.

Smits, Jasper A. J., Mark B. Powers, David Rosenfield, Michael J. Zvolensky, Jolene Jacquart, Michelle L. Davis, et al. 2016. "BDNF Val66Met Polymorphism as a Moderator of Exercise Enhancement of Smoking Cessation Treatment in Anxiety Vulnerable Adults." *Mental Health and Physical Activity* 10 (March): 73–77.

Snyder, C. R. 2000. *Handbook of Hope: Theory, Measures & Applications.* San Diego, CA: Academic Press.

Sprague, Jennifer E., and Ana María Arbeláez. 2011. "Glucose Counterregulatory Responses to Hypoglycemia." *Pediatric Endocrinology Reviews* 9(1): 463–475.

Stanczykiewicz, Bartlomiej, Anna Banik, Nina Knoll, Jan Keller, Diana Hilda Hohl, Joanna Rosinczuk, and Aleksandra Luszczynska. 2019. "Sedentary Behaviors and Anxiety Among Children, Adolescents, and Adults: A Systematic Review and Meta-Analysis." *BMC Public Health* 19 (1): 459.

Stipanuk, Martha H., and Yvonne Alexopolous. 2006. *Biochemical, Physiological & Molecular Aspects of Human Nutrition.* Second Edition. Philadelphia: Saunders.

Suliman, Sharain, Sian M. J. Hemmings, and Soraya Seedat. 2013. "Brain-Derived Neurotrophic Factor (BDNF) Protein Levels in Anxiety Disorders: Systematic Review and Meta-Regression Analysis." *Frontiers in Integrative Neuroscience* 7 (July): 55.

Sullivan Bisson, Alycia N., Stephanie A. Robinson, and Margie E. Lachman. 2019. "Walk to a Better Night of Sleep: Testing the Relationship between Physical Activity and Sleep." *Sleep Health* 5 (5): 487–494.

Vaucher, Paul, Pierre-Louis Druais, Sophie Waldvogel, and Bernard Favrat. 2012. "Effect of Iron Supplementation on Fatigue in Nonanemic Menstruating Women with Low Ferritin: A Randomized Controlled Trial." *CMAJ: Canadian Medical Association Journal* 184 (11): 1247–1254.

Verdon, F., B. Burnand, C. L. Fallab Stubi, C. Bonard, M. Graff, A. Michaud, et al. 2003. "Iron Supplementation for Unexplained Fatigue in Non-Anaemic Women: Double Blind Randomised Placebo Controlled Trial." *BMJ* 326 (7399): 1124.

Walker, Matthew P. 2017. *Why We Sleep: Unlocking the Power of Sleep and Dreams.* New York: Penguin.

Warren, Roderick E., and Brian M. Frier. 2005. "Hypoglycaemia and Cognitive Function." *Diabetes, Obesity & Metabolism* 7 (5): 493–503.

Watson, Nathaniel F., M. Safwan Badr, Gregory Belenky, Donald L. Bliwise, Orfeu M. Buxton, Daniel Buysse, et al. 2015. "Recommended Amount of Sleep for a Healthy Adult: A Joint Consensus Statement of the American Academy of Sleep Medicine and Sleep Research Society." *Sleep* 38 (6): 843–844.

Wild, Conor J., Emily S. Nichols, Michael E. Battista, Bobby Stojanoski, and Adrian M. Owen. 2018. "Dissociable Effects of Self-Reported Daily Sleep Duration on High-Level Cognitive Abilities." *Sleep* 41 (12): zsy182.

Withall, Janet, Russell Jago, and Kenneth R. Fox. 2011. "Why Some Do but Most Don't. Barriers and Enablers to Engaging Low-Income Groups in Physical Activity Programmes: A Mixed Methods Study." *BMC Public Health* 11 (June): 507.

Kristen Allott, ND, MS, is a naturopathic physician, national speaker, and pioneering advocate for the use of whole-foods nutrition in the treatment of mental health disorders and addictions. Allott is passionate about achievable results to improve energy, mental clarity, and decision-making. Drawing on her experience as a clinician, a wellness director for people in addiction recovery, a black belt in Aikido, and an advocate for individuals experiencing food insecurity, she helps people live better and more engaged lives.

Natasha Duarte, MS, is an innovative and inclusive advocate with proven success in building relationships with widely diverse people from multiple cultures. Her science background combined with strong social and cultural skills brings unique perspective to her work with food access, mental health, and building resilient communities. Duarte strongly believes that everyone should have the opportunity to be their best selves.

Foreword writer **Chan M. Hellman, PhD**, is internationally renowned for his work on building a hope-centered response to trauma. With over 150 scholarly publications and countless workshops in the areas of child maltreatment, domestic violence, homelessness, etc., Chan has focused his work on sharing the science and power of hope in our ability to overcome trauma and thrive.

Real change *is* possible

For more than forty-five years, New Harbinger has published proven-effective self-help books and pioneering workbooks to help readers of all ages and backgrounds improve mental health and well-being, and achieve lasting personal growth. In addition, our spirituality books offer profound guidance for deepening awareness and cultivating healing, self-discovery, and fulfillment.

Founded by psychologist Matthew McKay and Patrick Fanning, New Harbinger is proud to be an independent, employee-owned company. Our books reflect our core values of integrity, innovation, commitment, sustainability, compassion, and trust. Written by leaders in the field and recommended by therapists worldwide, New Harbinger books are practical, accessible, and provide real tools for real change.

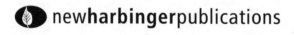 **newharbinger**publications

MORE BOOKS from
NEW HARBINGER PUBLICATIONS

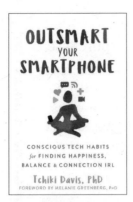
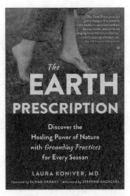
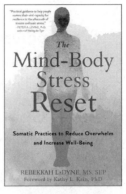
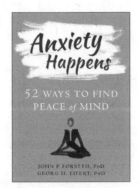
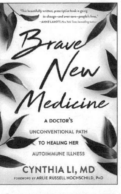
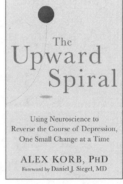
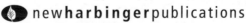

Register your **new harbinger** titles for additional benefits!

When you register your **new harbinger** title—purchased in any format, from any source—you get access to benefits like the following:

- Downloadable accessories like printable worksheets and extra content

- Instructional videos and audio files

- Information about updates, corrections, and new editions

Not every title has accessories, but we're adding new material all the time.

Access free accessories in 3 easy steps:

1. Sign in at NewHarbinger.com (or **register** to create an account).

2. Click on **register a book**. Search for your title and click the **register** button when it appears.

3. Click on the **book cover or title** to go to its details page. Click on **accessories** to view and access files.

That's all there is to it!

If you need help, visit:

NewHarbinger.com/accessories

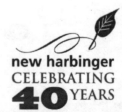

new harbinger
CELEBRATING
40 YEARS